POST-TRAUMATIC STRESS DISORDER:

ASSESSMENT, DIFFERENTIAL DIAGNOSIS, AND FORENSIC EVALUATION

EDITED BY
CARROLL L. MEEK, PhD

Professional Resource Exchange, Inc.
Sarasota, Florida

Hardbound Edition ISBN: 0-943158-35-4
Library of Congress Catalog Card Number: 89-43413

The production supervisor for this book was Debbie Fink,
the graphics coordinator was Laurie Girsch, and the cover
designer was Bill Tabler.

Dedication

This book is dedicated to all of those individuals who have suffered trauma, abuse, and disaster and who have contributed, thereby, in some way, to our understanding of the psychological torment they have experienced and their efforts and struggles to overcome the blows dealt to them. My hope is that we will become better providers of help to those injured.

This book is dedicated especially to my brother, Jon Bradley Larson, and my nephews, Jon Bradley Larson, Jr., and Michael David Larson, who did not survive the automobile accident that claimed them all, May 21, 1978.

> *"Hope is the thing with feathers -*
> *That perches in the soul -*
> *And sings the tune without the words -*
> *And never stops - at all.*
>
> *And sweetest - in the Gale - is heard -*
> *And sore must be the storm -*
> *That could abash the little Bird*
> *That kept so many warm -*
>
> *I've heard it in the chillest land -*
> *And on the strangest Sea -*
> *Yet, never, in Extremity,*
> *It asked a crumb - of Me."*

Emily Dickinson
c. 1861

*Note. Emily Dickinson (Poem #254) in The Complete Poems of Emily Dickinson (20th ed.) (p. 116) by T. H. Johnson (Ed.), 1960, Boston: Little, Brown & Co.

Acknowledgments

I would like to thank all of those who took time out of their busy days to research the literature and record their experience related to their assigned topics. My heartfelt gratitude goes to Herbert C. Modlin, MD, of the Menninger Clinic; Herbert J. Cross, PhD, of Washington State University; Cindy Miller-Perrin, MS, of Washington State University and Sandy Wurtele, PhD, of the University of Colorado; Emmett Early, PhD, in independent practice in Seattle, Washington; and Charles Z. Smith, JD, attorney in Seattle, Washington.

I would also like to acknowledge the Professional Resource Exchange, Inc., for encouraging this project and for the patience and support given when deadlines were extended and postponed. Thank you all!

Of course, in any undertaking like this there were others who were short-changed while we worked late-night hours to finish this book. Everyone on this page has someone who undoubtedly sacrificed as well. For those of you, unnamed, thank you, too.

I would like to thank my parents, Leland C. and Doris H. Larson, who I am sure sacrificed more than I will ever know for my education and suffered years of neglect while I steadfastly pursued it. To my husband, Saul M. Spiro, MD, who served as my research assistant and critic, I will be forever grateful. Although I could not persuade him to contribute a chapter to this volume, his expertise has served countless Washington State University students who have gone on to write their own books and to work in the clinical area with traumatized people. Besides, no one could possibly ask for a better companion.

Thank you, too, to "Katrina" who snuggles the closest to those who are the most deeply distressed, kisses away tears, and encourages some of the first smiles to emerge from depression and the memories of trauma . . . .

Table of Contents

Dedication   iii

Acknowledgments   v

List of Tables   xi

1. **Introduction**
   Carroll L. Meek   1

2. **Evaluation and Assessment of Post-
   Traumatic and Other Stress-Related Disorders**
   Carroll L. Meek   9

   Historical Summary   9
   Research Regarding Severe Stressors   10
   Determination of the Extent of the Stressors   12
   Assessment of the Psychological "Meaning" of the Stressors   13
   Compounding Factors in Stress-Related Mental Disorders   14
   Assessment of Additional Stress-Related Symptoms   17
   Variations in Reactions to Stress and Vulnerabilities   19
   Physical Injuries and Stress-Related Disorders   24
   Stress-Related Disorders in Individuals Not Exposed
        "Directly" to the Trauma   25
   Stress-Related Diagnoses   26
     Differential Diagnoses in Childhood and Adolescence   26
     Differential Diagnoses in Adulthood   30
   Grief and Bereavement as Possible Complications of
        Stress-Related Disorders   30
   Differential Diagnosis and Compounding Disorders That May Not Be
        Reactions to Specific or Identified Severe Stressors   40
   Testing   46
   Self-Evaluation of Difficulties Questionnaire   50
   References   52

3. **Post-Traumatic Stress Disorder: Differential Diagnosis**
   Herbert C. Modlin   63

   Generalized Anxiety Disorder   64
   Panic Disorder   65
   Major Depressive Episode   67
   Post-Concussion Syndrome   69
   References   72

4. **Social Factors Associated with Post-Traumatic
   Stress Disorder in Vietnam Veterans**
   Herbert J. Cross   73

   Description of Post-Traumatic Stress Disorder   75
   Problems with the Post-Traumatic Stress Disorder Concept   78
   Prevalence of Post-Traumatic Stress Disorder in Vietnam,
      Korean, and World War II Veterans   79
   The Vietnam Trauma   79
   The Post-Traumatic Stress Disorder-Resentment Continuum   82
   Forensic Application   85
   References   87

5. **Reactions to Childhood Sexual Abuse:
   Implications for Post-Traumatic Stress Disorder**
   Cindy L. Miller-Perrin and Sandy K. Wurtele   91

   Child Sexual Abuse   91
   Can Child Sexual Victimization Result in Harmful Effects?   92
      Initial Effects   93
         Clinical Studies   94
         Empirical Studies   96
      Long-Term Effects   100
         Clinical Samples   100
         Random Samples   104
         College Populations   104
         Summary   105
   Studies Suggesting a Relationship Between Childhood Sexual
      Trauma and Post-Traumatic Stress Disorder   105
   Post-Traumatic Stress Disorder in Young Sexual Abuse Victims   107
   Post-Traumatic Stress Disorder in Adults Abused as Children   112
   Implications   116
      Assessment   116
      Therapeutic Intervention   120
      Research Issues   123
   References   125

6. **Imagined, Exaggerated, and Malingered Post-Traumatic Stress Disorder**
   Emmett Early   137

   Differential Diagnosis   139
   Concurrent Disorders   143
   Exaggerating Post-Traumatic Stress Disorder   144
   Evaluation Problems   146
   Psychometric Evaluation   149
   Summary   151
   References   152

7. **Forensic Issues in Post-Traumatic Stress Disorder**
   Herbert C. Modlin   157

   Personal Injury Suits   158
   Workers' Compensation Claims   159
   Proximate Cause   160
   Predisposition   161
   Disability   162
   Reports   164
   Conclusion   166
   References   166

8. **Definitions, Procedures, and Guidelines for Expert Witnesses**
   Charles Z. Smith   167

   The Therapist as Witness   167
   The Federal Rules of Evidence   174
      Rule 611. Mode and Order of Interrogation and Presentation   175
      Rule 612. Writing Used to Refresh Memory   176
      Rule 613. Prior Statements of Witnesses   176
      Rule 614. Calling and Interrogation of Witnesses by Court   177
      Rule 615. Exclusion of Witnesses   177
      Rule 504. Psychotherapist-Patient Privilege (Proposed)   178
      Rule 701. Opinion Testimony By Lay Witnesses   183
      Rule 702. Testimony by Experts   183
      Rule 703. Bases of Opinion Testimony By Experts   183
      Rule 705. Disclosure of Facts or Data Underlying
              Expert Opinion   184
      Rule 104. Preliminary Questions   184
   Advice for the Therapist as Witness   191
   References   193

Appendix: Self-Evaluation of Difficulties Questionnaire
   Carroll L. Meek   197

Author Index   217

Subject Index   227

List of Tables

Table 2.1 Stress-Related Disorders: Compounding, Contributing, Causal, Associated, or Predisposing Factors   32

Table 2.2 Disorders That May Not be Due to Reactions to Specific or Extreme Stressors   47

Table 5.1 Initial Effects Reported Among Sexually Abused Children and Adolescents   95

Table 5.2 Long-Term Effects Reported Among Adults Sexually Abused as Children   101

Table 5.3 Classification of the Initial (I) and Long-Term (LT) Effects of Sexual Abuse According to Post-Traumatic Stress Disorder Criteria and Associated Symptoms   109

POST-TRAUMATIC
STRESS DISORDER:

ASSESSMENT, DIFFERENTIAL DIAGNOSIS,
AND FORENSIC EVALUATION

1.

Introduction

Carroll L. Meek

My research into the psychological and psychiatric literature regarding post-traumatic stress disorder (PTSD) was occasioned by a client who was referred to me by her physician because of the symptoms she was experiencing in the aftermath of a serious automobile accident in which she and several members of her family had been involved. She was evidencing constant associations to the event, had nighttime and daytime intrusive recollections of the accident, showed startle reactions, and was having difficulties answering the door and telephone. She also was having problems relating to her husband on an intimate level, was emotionally volatile, and was finding it difficult to fall asleep and remain asleep because of her nightmares. She felt enormous guilt regarding the fact that her family had been in this accident, although she had not been driving. She felt inordinately responsible for the problems her mother and infant might develop as a result of the accident. She also took emotional responsibility for her husband's physical injuries and resulting medical problems. She was not dealing well with ongoing obligations and was having difficulties finding the right words to express herself. She could not concentrate on a task long enough to carry it through to completion. She was avoiding more and more activities and experienced growing fears of driving, ultimately refusing to operate an automobile except in unusual circumstances.

Associations to the accident were increasing, especially when litigation became prolonged (lasting for years),

1

with no promise of settlement and no offer of financial assistance in the interim. In addition, employment possibilities narrowed for both husband and wife: for him because of his physical injuries and for her because of her emotional problems. Onset of her PTSD, which clearly met all diagnostic criteria specified in the third edition of the *Diagnostic and Statistical Manual of Mental Disorders (DSM-III*, American Psychiatric Association, 1980), and the revised third edition (*DSM-III-R*, American Psychiatric Association, 1987), was within 6 months of the trauma and clearly lasted longer than 6 months. Therefore, during the time I saw her in psychotherapy, the acute diagnosis of the disorder was changed to PTSD, chronic. Later, when it became obvious that in addition to the diagnosis of PTSD, she also met the criteria for major depression, that diagnosis was added.

The attorneys who had been retained to represent this family had built their case upon the pure and simple fact (for her) of the development of PTSD, which had been caused by the accident. When the diagnosis of major depression was made, they quickly settled the claim out of court, for a much smaller amount than that for which they had previously hoped. They settled, I believe, because they did not understand that the finding of major depression did not, in any way, negate the stress-induced PTSD response originally diagnosed as being caused by the automobile accident.

Although I felt I had thoroughly acquainted myself with the PTSD literature, I had been unable to demonstrate to the attorneys that there are many different responses, and associated diagnoses, that people might evidence as a result of severe or multiple stresses. I felt that the stress-related literature needed to be organized in some way so that people involved with stress-related diagnoses could understand that there are many implications and complications in this area.

It is important to demonstrate that PTSD is not the only diagnostically significant mental disorder possible as a response to a severe trauma or multiple traumas, but that other mental disorders can also develop in response to severe stressors. The clinician needs to be able to delineate how these diagnoses are derived, ruled out, or added as information becomes available regarding a particular individual's reaction to trauma and stresses - especially when these stresses and traumas are documentable events.

Because of the publicity regarding PTSD resulting from the Vietnam experience, it became clear that the attorneys believed it to be a viable diagnosis. It did not occur to these attorneys, perhaps because of the lack of equal publicity, that there are other stress-related disorders that are also significant. Because of this lack of media coverage and, therefore, of public awareness, it may be more difficult (but necessary) to convince the lay public that disorders other than PTSD might occur in the wake of severe traumas, and also can be incapacitating or diminish the individual's ability to function.

As stress-response groups are being identified and studied, it has become clear that varied responses to stress do occur. Also, as more information accumulates, it may become possible to predict who may be likely candidates for a stress-related disorder in terms of previous stresses, personality makeup, or co-existing mental pathologies.

The attorneys in this case were certainly not the only dubious individuals. Vietnam veterans faced doubt and professionals in the field have also expressed it. Dubiousness regarding stress-related diagnoses has been recent even among professionals. The following quotation is so poignant, it seemed logical to include it, at least as an indication of that to which the clinician must be prepared to respond - particularly when dealing with a lay population (i.e., attorneys, judges, juries, friends, co-workers, and relatives).

> Several years ago, at a professional meeting devoted to a discussion of victims of terrorism, a talented researcher presented her findings in regard to a group of children who had been buried alive for 24 hours [27 cited in Beigel & Berren, 1985, p. 147]. She had interviewed the children subsequent to the disaster and had spent time with their families and friends. She presented meticulously collected, carefully detailed historical and observational data of the psychiatric sequelae following this major disaster. She elaborated on the short-term and long-term responses of these stressed children in the process presenting hypothetical data about new defense mechanisms and post-traumatic stress in children. Although the paper was well-done, scholarly and fascinating, the reaction of the discussant, typically a mild-mannered, polite intellectual, was enraged. He

questioned the researcher's findings and accused her of overpsychologizing. The attending professional group of mental health experts enforced his denial of the effect of trauma and disaster on previously healthy children. The group became involved in a discussion of the research methodology, statistical tests vs. clinical observation and validity of data derived from play therapy. [It sounds like a court of law, does it not?] At first it seemed that the participants in the conference were not child psychiatrists and thus did not understand play therapy and how observational data about children could be derived from it. This distinctly unusual response with characteristics of hostility, rage and incredulity seemed to be a massive form of denial. This was but another manifestation of a long tradition of denying psychological and psychiatric sequelae in the child/victim of disaster. The audience response of disbelief in the face of carefully collected documentation of the presented data might have been so intense because it was difficult for *professionals* [emphasis mine] to accept the fact that a single highly traumatic event might color and shape the lives of these child/victims of disaster for at least 5 years.*

This research regarding the children of the Chowchilla school-bus kidnaping (July 15, 1976; Beigel & Berren, 1985) was published by Terr in 1979 and 1981 (cited in Benedek, 1985). Others have noted bias among professionals regarding the existence of the PTSD diagnosis as well (Atkinson et al., 1982).

The *DSM-III* did not mention PTSD in children, although the diagnosis was not specifically "excluded" as a diagnostic category for children. When the original form of this paper (Meek, 1985a, 1985b) was presented at the Expert Witness and Courtroom Testimony conference in Bellevue, Washington (September 13-14, 1985), sponsored by the Alternatives to Sexual Abuse organization, this diagnosis (where children were involved) seemed to have eluded some of the members of the audience (all profes-

---

sionals) even there. One therapist indicated that he had been treating a victim of the California McDonald's Restaurant shoot-out. The child, who was 6 years old at the time of the incident, was wounded, as was his father, and his mother and sister were both killed. After they moved to Washington State, his teacher there made a pointed effort to challenge this little boy about the accuracy of his report and indicated a profound belief that he had fabricated the entire incident. The absence of support in his new environment and the disbelief that this tragedy had even occurred worsened the child's emotional condition. The therapist was incredulous that his little patient had all of the symptoms of PTSD, yet he had never considered the diagnosis a possibility.

The following topics were selected for inclusion in this volume in an effort to help practitioners deal with particular problems that are likely to present themselves in any practice. It is hoped that the information will adequately inform or, at least, help them study those areas even more extensively and thoroughly.

Chapter 2, "Evaluation and Assessment of Post-Traumatic and Other Stress-Related Disorders" by Carroll L. Meek, PhD, was written to help professionals differentiate the types of difficulties and disorders that people experience as responses to multiple or severe stressors. The chapter also attempts to anticipate legal questions that might arise during the course of an investigation and, therefore, to help the practitioner provide thoughtful and well-researched answers.

Chapter 3, "Post-Traumatic Stress Disorder: Differential Diagnosis" by Herbert C. Modlin, MD, adeptly and simply addresses the issue of how clinicians differentiate several disorders from one another. Since questions arise in terms of why a clinician chooses one disorder over another when making a diagnosis, it behooves the clinician to address those issues by being able to point out the differences, if asked.

Chapter 4, "Social Factors Associated with Post-Traumatic Stress Disorder in Vietnam Veterans" by Herbert J. Cross, PhD, discusses special problems and issues involving this pivotal group. Due to the fact that Vietnam veterans experienced difficulties in such great numbers, the issue of PTSD resurfaced in the psychiatric nomenclature. Dr. Cross addresses some of the factors that continue to separate the Vietnam veteran from others who have experienced severe and/or multiple stressors.

Chapter 5. "Reactions to Childhood Sexual Abuse: Implications for Post-Traumatic Stress Disorder" by Cindy L. Miller-Perrin, MS, and Sandy K. Wurtele, PhD, addresses the difficulties experienced by another group that is also receiving more and more attention. With the emphasis on teaching children their rights to freedom from sexual abuse and with greater public awareness of this widespread problem, children are becoming more likely to speak out when having difficulties. In addition, women who were abused in the past continue to experience symptoms or develop disorders. Ms. Miller-Perrin and Dr. Wurtele skillfully address the particular and continuing problems of this group of traumatized people. They also offer implications for treatment and research in this area.

Chapter 6, "Imagined, Exaggerated, and Malingered Post-Traumatic Stress Disorder" by Emmett Early, PhD, outlines many of the problems and diagnostic strategies that need to be considered by the clinician who is confronted with individuals presenting difficulties because of trauma. As implied by the title, the clinician must, at the very least, explore the possibilities of these types of fabrication. When legal proceedings are instigated, the practitioner can or should assume that these potential problems will be addressed or questioned.

Chapter 7. "Forensic Issues in Post-Traumatic Stress Disorder" by Herbert C. Modlin, MD, outlines many of the concepts and situations practitioners need to expect from patients at some time during their practice. Dr. Modlin explores some of the legal questions the clinician must consider and delineates and simplifies points in law that are generally foreign to clinicians who are inexperienced in terms of the specific questions that must be answered and the legal definitions of the repercussions of injury or damage.

Finally, Chapter 8, "Definitions, Procedures, and Guidelines for Expert Witnesses" by Charles Z. Smith, JD, explores the legal expectations of the therapist as an expert witness. The author presents rules of evidence that are likely to be applicable to the circumstances in which therapists may find themselves when possessing confidential information about a client.

I hope that this volume will increase the clinician's expertise and familiarity in this complicated area.

Carroll L. Meek, PhD, has been in independent practice as a counseling psychologist since 1982. For 13 years prior to this, she was in Counseling Services at Washington State University, Pullman. She received her BA degree in psychology from Whitman College, Walla Walla, WA in 1964; her MS degree in student personnel in higher education from Indiana University, Bloomington, IN in 1966; and her PhD degree in guidance and counseling from the University of Idaho, Moscow, ID in 1972. In addition to her work at Washington State University, she was a counselor at the University of Idaho's Counseling Center for 1 year and was a counselor and head resident at the University of Wisconsin, Oshkosh, for 2 years. Dr. Meek may be contacted at The Professional Mall, S.E. 1205 Professional Mall Boulevard, Pullman, WA 99163.

REFERENCES

American Psychiatric Association. (1980). *Diagnostic and Statistical Manual of Mental Disorders* (3rd ed.). Washington, DC: Author.

American Psychiatric Association. (1987). *Diagnostic and Statistical Manual of Mental Disorders* (3rd ed. rev.). Washington, DC: Author.

Atkinson, R. M., Henderson, R. G., Sparr, L. F., & Deale, S. (1982, September). Assessment of Viet Nam veterans for posttraumatic stress disorder in veterans administration disability claims. *American Journal of Psychiatry, 139*, 1118-1121.

Beigel, A., & Berren, M. R. (1985, March). Human-induced disasters. *Psychiatric Annals, 15*, 143-144, 147-148, 150.

Benedek, E. D. (1985, March). Children and disaster: Emerging issues. *Psychiatric Annals, 15*, 168-172.

Meek, C. L. (1985a, September). *Post-Traumatic Stress Disorder Evaluation Form.* Unpublished manuscript presented at the Expert Witness and Courtroom Testimony Conference, sponsored by Alternatives to Sexual Abuse, Bellevue, WA.

Meek, C. L. (1985b, September). *Post-Traumatic Stress Disorder Evaluation of Personal Injury.* Paper presented at the Expert Witness and Courtroom Testimony Conference, sponsored by Alternatives to Sexual Abuse, Bellevue, WA.

2.

Evaluation and Assessment of Post-Traumatic and Other Stress-Related Disorders

Carroll L. Meek

HISTORICAL SUMMARY

A brief historical summary regarding the diagnosis of post-traumatic stress disorder (PTSD) needs to be included in any major survey of stress-related disorders, because it seems obvious that this disorder opened the door to a more realistic study of stress reactions in general. In addition, many clinicians will be required to respond to specific types of stressors. The literature involving the many situations in which these disorders have been identified and examined might prove to be helpful, especially since what exists as something "significant" enough to qualify as a stressor is open to argument from all sides. Readers studying various types of stressors may find the following literature review helpful.

Post-traumatic stress disorder has been known to professionals and others since the Civil War (Scrignar, 1987), World War I, and certainly World War II (Christenson et al., 1981; Corcoran, 1982; Hamilton & Canteen, 1987; Van Dyke, Zilberg, & McKinnon, 1985); and decidedly after the Vietnam conflict (Allen, 1986; Arnold, 1985; Atkinson et al., 1982; Atkinson et al., 1984; Blank, 1985; Boulanger, 1985; Braceland, 1982; Breslau & Davis, 1987; Friedman et al., 1986; Frye & Stockton, 1982; Garb, Bleich, & Lerer, 1987; Groesbeck, 1982; Hendin et al., 1981; Laufer, Brett, & Gallops, 1985; Lifton, 1982; Lipkin, Blank, & Scurfield, 1985; Pina, 1985; Scurfield & Blank, 1985; Shatan, 1982;

Silver, 1985; Singer, 1981; Smith, 1982; Sonnenberg, Blank, & Talbott, 1985; Ursano, 1981; Ursano, Boydstun, & Wheatley, 1981; Walker & Cavenar, 1982). Many viewed Vietnam veterans' problems with a great deal of skepticism for more than a decade (Braceland, 1982; Groesbeck, 1982). It was the Vietnam war, however, that apparently prompted PTSD's inclusion as a diagnostic category in the third edition of the *Diagnostic and Statistical Manual of Mental Disorders (DSM-III*, American Psychiatric Association, 1980; Ettedgui & Bridges, 1985). It was not until the *DSM-III* was published in 1980, that PTSD was once again acknowledged as a "mental disorder." That diagnosis was given in *DSM-I* under "gross stress reaction" (Andreasen, 1980) and was dropped completely from the *DSM-II*, apparently because of a peacetime lull when few war-related cases came to light (Andreasen, 1980).

The PTSD diagnosis has been called by many names, including traumatic neurosis, traumatic war neurosis, combat neurosis, combat fatigue, combat exhaustion, battle stress, operational fatigue (Andreasen, 1980), conversion hysteria (Cornfield & Hogben, 1980), and rape trauma syndrome (Burgess & Holmstrom, cited in Modlin, 1983).

RESEARCH REGARDING SEVERE STRESSORS

According to the *DSM-III*, the first criterion that was required in establishing the existence of PTSD was the "existence of a recognizable stressor that would evoke significant symptoms of distress in almost *everyone* [emphasis mine]" (p. 238). This has been qualified in the *DSM-III-R* to "an event that is outside the range of usual human experience and that would be markedly distressing to almost *anyone* [emphasis mine]" (p. 250). "Almost *everyone*" has been changed to "almost *anyone*" - thereby paving the way to the recognition that stressors may affect individuals differently.

Assessment, necessarily, involves discussion of the stressor itself. Some may argue with what is or is not a significant stressor, so it becomes important to determine whether the stressor is outside the realm of "usual human experience." Usual experiences are considered to include the loss of a job, chronic illness, marital difficulties, divorce, and the like. However, research cited later in this chapter will indicate that these problems, coupled with severe stressors or multiple stressors, may compound the individual's psychological situation accordingly.

Situations or stressors that are considered to be outside the realm of usual human experiences include participating in war and combat (Allen, 1986; Archibald et al., 1962; Friedman et al., 1986; Lavie et al., 1979; Levav, Greenfeld, & Baruch, 1979; Shatan, 1982; Silver, 1985; Solomon & Benbenishty, 1986; Solomon et al., 1987a; Solomon et al., 1987b; Wilmer, 1982); being held in a prisoner-of-war camp (Arthur & McKenna, 1982; Boehnlein et al., 1985; Hall & Malone, 1976; Singer, 1981; Tennant, Goulston, & Dent, 1986; Ursano et al., 1981); being held hostage (Hillman, 1981); fires (Andreasen, 1980, McFarlane, 1986); being involved in collisions at sea or marine explosions (Hoiberg & McCaughey, 1984; Leopold & Dillon, 1963); suffering rape and sexual assault or abuse (Burgess & Holmstrom, 1974; Finkelhor, 1987; Fox & Scherl, 1972; Jackson, Quevillon, & Petretic-Jackson, 1985; Nadelson et al., 1982; Notman & Nadelson, 1976; Rose, 1986; Santiago et al., 1985); undergoing physical trauma (Ravenscroft, 1982); being a victim of incest (Lindberg & Distad, 1985); witnessing the torture of other people or being a worker on an extremely distressing scene involving mutilated, dead, or anguished individuals (Arnold, 1985; Arthur & McKenna, 1983; Breslau & Davis, 1987; McKenna & Arthur, 1983; Rothschild, 1984; Silver, 1985; Wilkinson & Vera, 1985); being parents or other relatives of victims (Benedek, 1985; Erikson, 1976; Lindy, 1985; Rangell, 1976; Ravenscroft, 1982; Rothschild, 1984; Stern, 1976; Wilkinson & Vera, 1985); experiencing the death of a close friend or relative (Haley, 1985); being a prisoner in a concentration camp (Boehnlein et al., 1985; Corcoran, 1982; Dimsdale, 1974; Eaton, Sigal, & Weinfeld, 1982; Kinzie et al., 1984); and undergoing those experiences that result from natural disasters and disasters caused by acts of human omission, commission, or recklessness (Beigel & Berren, 1985; Erikson, 1976; Lindy, 1985; Newman, 1976; Rangell, 1976; Shore, Tatum, & Vollmer, 1986; Stern, 1976; Titchener & Kapp, 1976; Wilkinson, 1983).

In the *DSM-III*, specific stressors mentioned that could be significant enough to produce symptoms of distress in almost everyone included rape or assault, military combat, floods, earthquakes, car accidents with serious physical injury, airplane crashes, large fires, bombing, torture, death camps, physical consequences or complications of the trauma (which included malnutrition and head injury), and so forth. In the *DSM-III-R*, largely because of the wealth of research that has been conducted in this area, the types of stressors that are considered to be "outside the range of usual human experience and that would be markedly distressing to almost anyone" (p. 250) have been expanded. In addition to the examples of stressors in the *DSM-III*, the following have been added in the *DSM-III-R*: receiving threats to one's life or "physical integrity" (p. 247) or to one's children, partner, or other close individuals; suffering the loss of one's home or community (including sudden loss or destruction); viewing another person who has been (or is being) killed or harmed (either accidentally or by deliberate physical violence); and learning about serious threats or harm to someone close (the *DSM-III-R* cites as an example that one has learned that "one's child has been kidnapped, tortured, or killed," p. 248).

DETERMINATION OF THE
EXTENT OF THE STRESSORS

It is important for the clinician to examine the existence of the stressor and its extent, although the final determination of emotional harm may be made by a legal system in cases that involve litigation (Hoffman, 1986). This reduces the burden of proof for the clinician in that regard, but an attempt to determine the range of traumatic events that could be included in "usual human experience" or that which most people might expect normally to experience sometime in their lifetime is necessary.

The *DSM-III-R* attempts to provide the clinician assistance in this regard with the inclusion of a more formal assessment list in the Severity of Psychosocial Stressors Scale for Adults and another for children and adolescents (*DSM-III-R*, p. 11) and the Global Assessment of Functioning Scale (GAF Scale, p. 12 - with instructions for using these scales appearing on pp. 18-20). The *DSM-III-R* suggests that in evaluating the stressors one should consider the following: (a) the extent of the change incurred in the person's life that apparently was caused by the stressor; this may be determined more easily by comparing circumstances or activities preceding the stressor with those occurring after it; (b) which aspects of the event were and were not under the person's control; and (c) the number of stressors - these, evidently, may be stressors occurring conjointly or they may be previous stressors endured by the individual, although this is not specifically delineated in the *DSM-III-R*. When rating the severity of the stressor, the *DSM-III-R* indicates that the clinician's determination should be based on the stressor and not on the person's vulnerability in that regard. However, the person's vulnerability is assessed elsewhere, particularly if the vulnerability includes another mental or personality disorder. The stressor should also be specified as acute (lasting less than 6 months) or enduring (lasting more than 6 months).

The *DSM-III-R* indicates that the determination regarding acute and enduring stressors may be diagnostically significant in that there is a tendency or a likelihood of differential responses to duration of a stressor. There also appears to be evidence that children might be at a greater risk for the development of a mental disorder following enduring stressors, with the implication that there may be a greater likelihood of adjustment to acute events.

The *DSM-III-R* encourages clinicians to denote more than one severe stressor, if more than one exists, but rarely are more than the four most severe stressors noted. When rating the severity of the stressors, the highest stressor's rating should be given and provision made for an increase in the rating if there are many stressors.

In addition to the traumas that are specifically mentioned for people with a diagnosis of a stress-related disorder, there are other types of psychosocial stress that can occur. The American Psychiatric Association (1987) proposes that the clinician investigate the following categories: conjugal (marital and nonmarital), parenting, other interpersonal problems, occupational, living circumstances, financial, legal, developmental, physical illness or injury, and family factors (for children and adolescents). Although not mentioned as an area of scrutiny for adults, in extended families the family factors mentioned might also be included as possible additional psychosocial stressors for adults, as well.

ASSESSMENT OF THE PSYCHOLOGICAL "MEANING" OF THE STRESSORS

According to many researchers, it is important to assess the meaning the stressor has had to the individual (Hendin et al., 1981; Leopold & Dillon, 1963; Lifton, 1982; Newman, 1976; Taylor, 1983; West & Coburn, 1984). In terms of losses, the literature indicates that these also include psychic losses. The person may have lost a sense of personal "invulnerability," and may feel that the environment and the people in it are no longer friends upon whom the person can depend. The world, for that person, may have become unreliable. Therefore, it is important for the clinician to inquire about how the person's perception of the world and the way it works has changed or seems different. There is evidence that the meanings a person assigns to the world and to the events may contribute to the exacerbation of a stress-related disorder. Garb and his associates (1987) cite losses of loved or valued friends, aspects of oneself, body parts, or function (including drives and interests), positive definitions of oneself, external objects, and developmental losses. They indicate that these losses are real as well as perceptual (i.e., they contain personal or symbolic meaning).

COMPOUNDING FACTORS IN
STRESS-RELATED MENTAL DISORDERS

This section will explore the compounding factors that might be involved because of severe trauma or other stressors. Although the disorders specifically addressed are mentioned in the *DSM-III-R* as disorders that can be responses to stresses, there are few in which the existence of specific types of stressors is required for the diagnosis to be made. When this condition is specified, it will, of course, be mentioned. However, it is important to note that individuals may develop any number of psychological disorders as a response to extreme stress (either because of the extreme nature of a stressor or of the existence of multiple stressors that may be less severe if taken individually).

The clinician should be alert to individual's idiosyncratic responses to stress. In addition, it should be noted that many people suffer from psychiatric disorders without ever making the association that their difficulties stem from particular stresses or trauma (Foy et al., 1987; Lindberg & Distad, 1985; Scrignar, 1987). Some cases have been diagnosed so many years after the original trauma, and the symptoms have been so far removed from the original stressor in time, that the individual does not mention any stressor or trauma as a probable cause of the symptoms (Horowitz, 1985). People evidencing symptoms of the *DSM-III-R* diagnostic criteria, especially those who mention the prior existence of a severe stressor, should be carefully questioned about previous stresses and painful experiences. Unless carefully questioned, the presence of guilt and lack of trust regarding therapy and evaluation may create an impasse in which the individual, rather than provoking previous painful memories, may drop out of therapy, refuse treatment, or refuse to continue with the evaluation. This lack of cooperation may be frustrating to the clinician and, indeed, a high percentage of individuals with extreme stress-related disorders refuse to proceed with therapy and other procedures designed to try to help them recover (Foy et al., 1987).

For those who are able to associate the beginning of their difficulties with their reaction to specific traumas, it seems likely that physicians or attorneys might be the first to be consulted regarding the onset of their symptoms or difficulties. Modlin (1967) mentioned that personal injury litigation might lead attorneys to be the first to identify or suspect the existence of PTSD or other stress-related disorders. If the person is involved in litigation regarding an act of omission or commission, the defense attorney can help the case by settling claims as quickly as possible (Andreasen, 1980; McKenna & Arthur, 1983). The reason for this is not that compensation claims, once settled, cause symptoms to disappear; they may not (Thompson, 1965). Research indicates that many cases of PTSD, in particular, are of the delayed or chronic type (Andreasen, 1980; Archibald et al., 1962; Beigel & Berren, 1985; Leopold & Dillon, 1963; Lindberg & Distad, 1985; Singer, 1981; Titchener & Kapp, 1976; among others). Therefore, the longer litigation continues and the greater the passage of time, the greater the likelihood that residual or delayed categories of PTSD and other stress-related disorders may either arise or be identified. In addition, the likelihood is also greater that chronicity will be demonstrated to be an ongoing problem that is not going to be cured by time alone.

The more chronic the symptoms are, the longer they last, or the more serious and complicated the loss or injury is, the worse is the prognosis for recovery or the longer the reaction time may be (Andreasen, 1980; Horowitz, 1985, 1986; Lifton, 1982; Schnaper & Cowley, 1976). Researchers have indicated that the longer a problem continues, the longer it is likely to continue - and this refers to stress reactions and mental disorders specifically

(Horowitz, 1986; Modlin, 1983). Horowitz (1986) emphasized early intervention for these very reasons.

Andreasen (1980) has indicated that PTSD may be triggered by increased stresses. She cites returning to work, increased responsibilities, or resuming activities as contributing factors. Other authors have included work, family, or academic pressures (Boehnlein et al., 1985; Kolb & Mutalipassi, 1982; Wilmer, 1982). Still others have pointed out that any stress may reactivate symptoms (Kinzie et al., 1984); as might events resembling the original trauma coupled with the aging process (Christenson et al., 1981) and subsequent life events (McFarlane, 1986). Christenson and associates cite the fact that losses associated with "involutional age, including parental loss, children leaving home, pending retirement, and increasing medical disabilities all serve as stressors that may reactivate a latent traumatic stress disorder" (p. 985). Cornfield and Hogben (1980) indicated that chronic states show "a deterioration over time rather than spontaneous improvement" (p. 5); others have made similar observations (Archibald et al., 1962; Boulanger, 1985; Eaton et al., 1982; Leopold & Dillon, 1963).

In addition, PTSD and other stress-related disorders may be exacerbated by concurrent traumas (Hoffman, 1986) or by stressors occurring in late life or in the aging process (Allen, 1986; Andreasen, 1980; Atkinson et al., 1982; Friedman et al., 1986; Wilkinson & Vera, 1985; Wilmer, 1982). Therefore, the longer the patient waits for claims to be settled or injuries to mend (psychologically or physically), the more likely it will be that additional stressors will enter into the life of the patient. The person may deal with additional stressors less adequately than before a trauma and this provides the clinician with the additional obligation to investigate whether further "losses of function" have occurred because of pre-existing mental disorders that might have been stressed further or have been exacerbated because of an identifiable stressor. It behooves the clinician to assess premorbid personality functioning and other factors so that changes or evidence of deterioration can be addressed, specifically, in this regard. As will be explored in greater detail, pre-existing personality disorders may render a person more vulnerable to stress-related disorders (Hoffman, 1986; Horowitz, 1986; Scrignar, 1987).

The stress of litigation itself, as well as unpaid bills and financial deterioration, also begin to be generalized into reminders of the traumatic event, and become secondarily associated with the trauma or assault - this increases the possibility that more and more accumulative events will become triggers or reminders of the painful event. Fears or terrors are similar feelings, regardless of whether they are prompted by events resembling the original trauma, or are now additional (or secondary) traumas such as having to face a courtroom and all that those uncertainties and lack of procedural familiarity may represent.

Researchers are now reporting that large-scale or mass disasters cause individuals to suffer from a "loss of communality" or loss of community. Erikson (1976) stated, "It is difficult for people to recover from the effects of individual trauma when the community on which they have depended remains [or becomes] fragmented" (p. 302). Rangell (1976) and Wilkinson and Vera (1985) alluded to the same loss. The continuity of support systems has been cited as a factor related to recovery (Horowitz, 1986).

ASSESSMENT OF ADDITIONAL STRESS-RELATED SYMPTOMS

Although not required by the *DSM-III* for diagnosis of PTSD, additional symptoms are often present in many individuals evidencing stress-related disorders, and some are now included in the *DSM-III-R* as part of the criteria for PTSD. These include the presence of greater irritability or angry outbursts. The person may also be more sporadic in emotional responses, unpredictable, or aggressive toward friends, family members, or strangers, with little or no provocation.

The second is the presence of impulsivity. It is not uncommon for individuals with PTSD to take sudden trips, move out of the country, be absent without explanation from their homes or jobs, change residence, or alter lifestyles in radical ways. It is important to assess for irritability, aggressivity (Modlin, 1983), and impulsivity (Andreasen, 1980), because these criteria are also mentioned in the diagnostic classification of antisocial personality disorder. These elements are also extremely common in those with PTSD, but were not present to a great degree prior to the extreme stressor. However, there is growing evidence that individuals with personality disorders (including antisocial personality disorder) may be more susceptible to stress-related disorders.

17

Third, the person may complain of or demonstrate emotional lability, autonomic lability (i.e., shakiness, jitteriness, palpitations, etc.), headaches, or vertigo (i.e., dizziness or giddiness). If any of these symptoms are present, it becomes important to rule out the existence of organic mental disorders or brain syndromes (Horowitz, 1986; Scrignar, 1987). The *DSM-III-R* repeatedly cautions either that the possibility of organic mental disorders be eliminated as causative factors of symptoms that might also be present in stress-related disorders or that an organic mental disorder be diagnosed in conjunction with the stress disorder, if it seems likely that the organic mental disorder is not the sole cause of the stress-related symptoms. It is also important to consult with the individual's primary physician to determine whether any of the symptoms might be present because of a co-existent physiological trauma or injury (Andreasen, 1980; Dunn, 1981; Hoffman, 1986; Schnaper & Cowley, 1976; Thompson, 1965). If the physician suspects neurological trauma, referral to a neurologist or neuropsychologist may be indicated. Horowitz (1986) indicated that malnutrition can lead to organic brain syndromes and that concussions may have a long-term effect on mood.

Fourth, if the person is avoiding events or activities or is restricting his or her previous world, it is important to ascertain the events or situations that are being avoided. Phobic avoidance is not uncommon (Andreasen, 1980; Thompson, 1965; Wilkinson & Vera, 1985). Self-imposed restrictions as protection against further adverse emotional or psychic reactions are extremely common.

Fifth, one should determine whether relationships are deteriorating. One may wish to confer with spouse, children, neighbors, employers, or ministers regarding post-trauma changes they have observed in the individual. In addition to concerned family members and relatives, it is generally a good idea to interview at least one outside individual who knows the person well. Contrary to popular opinion, such individuals are good observers of changes in behavior. When litigation is involved, it can be argued that relatives and spouses of persons who have stress-related disorders have an equal or obvious stake in the outcome of the litigation. They, therefore, might be suspected to be biased observers, despite the adequacy or accuracy of their observations. Thus, a family friend or co-worker who is likely to be in a good position to be a reliable observer and is less likely to be a co-stress participant may be an important adjunct in determining behavioral, occupational, or relational changes post-stress.

VARIATIONS IN REACTIONS TO STRESS AND VULNERABILITIES

Although many researchers have stated that the PTSD syndrome "holds together" and is documentable (Atkinson et al., 1984; Boulanger, 1985; Ettedgui & Bridges, 1985; Thompson, 1965), questions regarding the legal implications in the assessment of PTSD and other stress-related disorders in personal injury cases arise, particularly when compensation is involved. The clinician must be apprised of all sides of these questions in order to avoid confusion, especially when called upon to serve as an expert witness.

The comment in the 1980 *DSM-III* under the subheading "Predisposing Factors" to the effect that "Preexisting psychopathology apparently predisposes to the development of the disorder" (referring specifically to PTSD, p. 337) also appeared elsewhere (Andreasen, 1980; Schottenfeld & Cullen, 1985 [atypical PTSD]; Thompson, 1965). Research on these predisposing factors now rests on evidence that it might be more likely that previous stress magnifies current stress, and that some personalities are either stronger, less inherently vulnerable, or "healthier" than others. Evidence is accumulating that some people are rendered more vulnerable because of the accumulation of stressors, pre-existing mental disorders, and personality factors. Because of the growing research documenting these greater vulnerabilities in some individuals, it is no longer necessary either to argue with these assumptions or to have to defend them.

Others (Atkinson et al., 1984; Burgess & Holmstrom, 1974; Lipkin et al., 1985) found no difference in prestressor symptoms and actual stressors among those with stress-related disorders and those without them. Fox and Scherl (1972), in their study of rape victims, found that their victims' past histories demonstrated "psychological health and achievement" (p. 37). Hall and Malone (1976) stated that "psychiatric symptoms are best viewed as normal reactions to abnormal situations" (p. 789). Hoiberg and McCaughey (1984) stated that the "major contributing factor to . . . psychological impairment was the disaster and not a history of mental disorders" (p. 72). Hoiberg and McCaughey also indicated that personal or demographic characteristics did not "predispose the men to post-

19

traumatic psychological impairment" (p. 72). Horowitz (1985) stated: "It should never be assumed, however, that a person who has developed a mental disorder after a disaster is a person who was a more impaired member of the population exposed to it" (p. 166). Lavie and associates (1979) did not find that PTSD individuals had been hospitalized, received psychiatric treatments, or suffered sleep impairment prior to their war experiences. Leopold and Dillon (1963) said that "the nature of the accident itself is a more significant determinant of post-traumatic psychological illness than the pre-accident personality; that such illness, if untreated, tends to worsen with time; and that litigation worries are a minor factor producing the illness" (p. 921). Also, Modlin (1967) noted that "symptoms vary negligibly from patient to patient and the precipitating stress looms large in any etiological explanation" (p. 1011). Nadelson and her associates (1982) found no history of mental or emotional disturbance in victims. The "preexisting vulnerabilities in the hosts to receive the invading organisms are not an issue" (Rangell, 1976, p. 314).

Shatan (1982) observed that "pre-existing psychiatric disorder is irrelevant" (p. 1035) when massive stress is present. Singer (1981) stated "the severity of the stresses imposed . . . are of more importance than predisposing personality factors in the development of poststress psychiatric disturbance" (p. 345). The results of work by Ursano and his associates (1981) "support the importance of the severity of the stress rather than predisposing personality factors in the development of poststress psychiatric disorder" and the researchers added that the "presence of psychiatric illness or predisposition to psychiatric illness is neither necessary nor sufficient for the illness after repatriation" (p. 315). Silver (1985) has aptly pointed out that the *DSM-III* diagnosis of PTSD did not "require" the existence of prior pathology; neither does that in the *DSM-III-R*. The *DSM-III-R* has added a sentence to the "Predisposing Factors" section in the discussion of PTSD that this disorder can occur in individuals who have not evidenced any pre-existing conditions, especially if there has been an "extreme stressor." The *DSM-III-R* also indicates that studies have found that pre-existing conditions are predispositions to the development of PTSD.

After evaluating the literature on PTSD, it became clear that even physically and psychologically normal people with no previous history of psychological disorder can develop characteristic responses to extreme stress (Atkinson et al., 1984; Bailey, 1985; Burgess & Holmstrom, 1974; Fox & Scherl, 1972; Hall & Malone, 1976; Hoiberg & McCaughey, 1984; Horowitz, 1985; Leopold & Dillon, 1963; Lipkin et al., 1985; Nadelson et al., 1982; Rangell, 1976; Shatan, 1982; Singer, 1981; Ursano et al., 1981). Since this is true, it also stands to reason that individuals who have experienced multiple previous traumas of varying intensities and those who have had prior emotional or psychological difficulties also would not be immune to additional traumas or extreme stressors (Beigel & Berren, 1985; Burgess & Holmstrom, 1974; Modlin, 1967, 1983).

Furthermore, it must be even more apparent in light of additional research in this area that any prior disorder that is exacerbated and caused to flare into even greater physical or emotional pain, discomfort, or torment is still grounds for damages to be awarded to the victim of trauma who suffers from PTSD or another stress-related disorder that arises because of an extreme stressor. Therefore, the clinician must include any exacerbations of previous conditions that might have been caused by an extreme stressor:

> . . . predisposition to neurotic breakdown is seldom considered relevant to the legal problems at hand. The law of torts states that the tortfeasor is equally liable if the injury caused the disability, activated a latent condition, or worsened a preexisting condition. As Justice Holmes observed, "The law is not for the physically sound alone." (Modlin, 1983, p. 680)

Hoffman (1986, p. 168) alludes to this as the "thin skull principle" (i.e., the defendant must take the victim as is and compensate for changes). If this were not the case, then a person who falls while playing volleyball and breaks an arm, and a week later is involved in the collapse of a hotel skywalk, suffers further abuse and trauma (e.g., concussion, broken leg, ankle, finger, or the other arm, or witnessing the death or injury of those who accompanied him or her) would fall victim to the reasoning that since he or she appeared to be doing quite well with the broken arm, then should not he or she also do well with these additional assaults to his or her person, and not be demonstrating symptoms of PTSD, depression, or anxiety?

Some researchers have indicated that rather than demonstrating that prior trauma or personality disorder excuses culpability in additional assaults, it may make ongoing assaults even more traumatic (Modlin, 1983; Wilkinson & Vera, 1985). Stress researchers have surmised that rather than traumas being dealt with serially, they may be cumulative in their impact (Beigel & Berren, 1985; Burgess & Holmstrom, 1974; Modlin, 1983; Shealy, 1984). Thus, the clinician must specifically ascertain whether the victim has suffered previous traumas and catastrophic events in his or her life, as well. The question is, "How much is the ordinary person likely to be able to stand?" Perhaps every person has a breaking point. One can assume that each individual may have a different point. Each person brings prior personalities and previous experiences into any event (Horowitz, 1985), and despite the efforts of researchers to pinpoint, precisely, what these events are likely to be, they may have been unable to demonstrate causes of stress-related disorders that are greater than specific stressors or rule them out. Van der Kolk (1987) indicated that that which overwhelms one person might not have the same impact on another and that childhood physical or sexual trauma may be a predisposing factor in the development of mental conditions in later years. He includes borderline personality disorder, multiple personality disorder, panic disorder, and chronic pain syndromes. Muse (1986) also cites chronic pain syndrome occurring as a result of physical trauma and that, coupled with life-threatening aspects of the trauma, is enough to precipitate PTSD in a large percentage of this particular population.

Preparedness and special training for crisis situations seem to be factors in the development of stress-related disorders. However, Leopold and Dillon (1963) indicated that long-term involvement in hazardous occupations dulls the person's capacity for "anticipation" of disaster - a factor in "preparedness." Anticipation of harm or injury apparently helps people deal with disasters. On the other hand, living with the actualities of automobile crashes and airline disasters, causes people to disregard the possibilities of accidents happening to themselves, because they occur so "infrequently." Betrayals in this respect make it more difficult to assimilate psychologically (McKenna & Arthur, 1983). Unexpectedness of trauma is likely to be critical in the development of stress-related disorders (Modlin, 1985; Notman & Nadelson, 1976). In addition, the absence of preparation or training seems to be related to the development of stress-related disorders (Bloch, 1978; Levav et al., 1979; West & Coburn, 1984).

In consideration of the factors that may contribute to the development of stress-related disorders, therefore, it is important to take a history of other traumatic events in the individual's life. Obtaining a history of social, educational, military, occupational, and vocational functioning (before and after a trauma) is necessary. In addition, medical and marital histories should be obtained (Andreasen, 1980; Arnold, 1985; Bailey, 1985; Lipkin et al., 1985; Modlin, 1967; Scurfield & Blank, 1985).

Although it is also important to assess previous psychopathology in the individual, because it may contribute to the development of stress-related disorders, it has already been emphasized that many individuals suffering from symptoms of a stress-related disorder may have been previously healthy, both psychologically and physically, and that previous pathology is not "required" for the diagnosis of PTSD (Silver, 1985) or other stress-related disorders. If additional psychopathology exists, however, it is necessary to assess, diagnose, and include those illnesses in a total evaluation if they have been exacerbated as a result of a stressor. Modlin (1983) presented the "chain of events" concept: "If the accident set off a chain of events beyond the capacity of the patient to control, the original tortfeasor may be held responsible for the outcome" (p. 679).

In fact, many of these comments regarding the victim's prior psychological or physical health and predisposing vulnerabilities may have been inspired by the legal defenses' tendency to argue against a patient's (plaintiff's) evidence of losses following a traumatic event in which litigation ensued, especially when pre-existing pathology could be demonstrated. That is similar to and probably is related to the insinuations often made in courts of law that a sexual assault victim's previous sexual history could somehow have had something to do with the occurrence of a traumatic event over which the victim actually had no control. Although the argument lacks much credibility, it is still used. Finkelhor (1987) has found that sexual victimization in childhood may lead to a higher risk of sexual victimization in the future - this would appear to create more vulnerability in those individuals, for reasons that are, so far, little understood.

Answers to many of the questions asked of clinicians serving in the capacity of expert witnesses may be confused if the motivations for the questions are unclear: "The individual seemed to be functioning extremely well, before now. Why is he or she now presenting these symptoms?" Evidence and understanding of the "previously healthy" and "predisposing vulnerabilities" literature can help the clinician answer these questions (i.e., nature of the stressor, multiple previous traumas, concurrent difficulties, etc.). "Since the individual obviously has had many previous difficulties functioning, how can you attribute these greater problems to this particular disaster?" Answering, again from the literature, the clinician can address the problem regarding pre-existing vulnerabilities (i.e., mental disorders, developmental problems, personality disorders, etc.) as possible contributing factors to a stress-related disorder and exacerbation of symptoms because of a lower tolerance to stresses, in particular.

PHYSICAL INJURIES AND STRESS-RELATED DISORDERS

Physical injury incurred during a trauma has been mentioned in the literature as likely to exacerbate PTSD and other stress-related disorders. It seems logical to assume that physical injury would magnify stress. In addition to fears and situations not under the individual's control, the person also has the physical pain, discomfort, or possibility of a disability that might last indefinitely (Andreasen, 1980). In addition to head trauma or concussion, the *DSM-III*, the *DSM-III-R*, and Horowitz (1986) mention malnutrition as a complicating factor. Horowitz associates malnutrition as a likely complication that may lead to organic brain syndromes - particularly during periods of prolonged stress - and indicates that concussions may also have a long-term effect on mood.

Archibald and his associates (1962) indicate that although physical injuries may reduce the individual's capacity to respond to stress, they may or may not exacerbate PTSD. However, Muse (1986) believes that the exacerbation hypothesis may be more likely to be true (i.e., life-threatening injuries coupled with chronic pain syndrome actually create greater risk for the subsequent development of PTSD).

Demonstrating the multiplicity of responses to stress, researchers have also found that those experiencing a catastrophic event who later exhibit symptoms of stress-related disorders may have had greater psychological

24

difficulties if they were not injured physically (Hoiberg & McCaughey, 1984; Modlin, 1983; Rothschild, 1984). The existence of physical injury may actually reduce the possibility of psychological disability (Modlin, 1983). It is puzzling as to why this might occur. It may be that a severe physical injury that people can see and objectively assess for themselves automatically leads to a stronger belief that the individual is, in fact, truly "injured," resulting in more frequent offers of assistance, greater empathy, and support. Support from others has already been cited as helping people recover more quickly from traumas (Horowitz, 1986).

STRESS-RELATED DISORDERS IN INDIVIDUALS NOT EXPOSED "DIRECTLY" TO THE TRAUMA

The recognition by the *DSM-III-R* of the possibility of stress responses of PTSD in people who have not been personally threatened during the trauma, or who may not have been present, is a result of the many studies that have been conducted since the *DSM-III* was published in 1980. This recognition is evident in the added examples of extreme situations that would be distressing to almost "anyone," such as learning about threats of or harm to another person (children, partner, close individuals), losing one's home or "community," or seeing something horrible happen to another person (the *DSM-III-R* cites the possibility or actuality of something horrible happening to one's child).

The Buffalo Creek Dam disaster studies fit into this category. Before this disaster, most legal judgments required that the victim had to have been victimized personally and directly in a severe way. This disaster was the first case in which people not actually present at the time the sludge (which was accumulated by a mining company) broke away and destroyed an entire community were awarded financial compensation (Stern, 1976). Six hundred and twenty-five individuals were awarded $13.5 million for losses, $6 million of which was for psychological damages, including "loss of community" - that which was known and relied upon in the course of everyday life (Stern, 1976). Research is indicating that rescuers at scenes of severe disasters also suffer adverse effects, and may even qualify for the diagnosis of PTSD or some other stress-related disorder (Arnold, 1985; Arthur &

McKenna, 1983; McKenna & Arthur, 1983; Rothschild, 1984; Silver, 1985; Wilkinson & Vera, 1985).

STRESS-RELATED DIAGNOSES

Since the *DSM-III-R* indicates that PTSD includes symptoms of depression and anxiety in many people, the existence of these disorders should be assessed. It is not unusual for people to develop an anxiety, depressive, or organic mental disorder after the occurrence of a significant stressor (Arnold, 1985; Atkinson et al., 1982). If they meet the criteria for any of these disorders, the diagnosis should be added to the diagnostic category of PTSD (American Psychiatric Association, 1987). Adjustment disorder, by definition, takes place in response to a less severe stressor than those required for the diagnosis of PTSD or reactive psychosis. Horowitz (1986) stated that adjustment disorder should not be regarded as a "minor disorder" (p. 245).

It is becoming quite clear that individuals develop many responses after experiencing an extreme trauma or multiple traumas. In addition, they may develop extreme responses to lesser traumas, particularly when there are pre-existing vulnerabilities or other mental or personality disorders. This makes it necessary for the clinician to determine whether patients have developed diagnosable conditions other than PTSD or in addition to PTSD following any specified stressor. If a person meets all the criteria for PTSD, that should be the diagnosis. If not, the person should be assessed for the existence of other mental disorders that might have arisen in response to the specified stressors.

In addition to PTSD, therefore, several other mental disorders may be stress related. Also, further evidence has indicated that personality disorders also need to be assessed because they may contribute to the individual's vulnerability to and adaptive capacity following stressors.

DIFFERENTIAL DIAGNOSES IN CHILDHOOD AND ADOLESCENCE

Since diagnostic categories were overlooked by clinicians with regard to children because of the lack of specific reference to them in previous diagnostic manuals, the *DSM-III-R* specifically cautions clinicians at the outset of the chapter titled "Disorders Usually First Evident in Infancy, Childhood, or Adolescence" that, in addition to the disorders mentioned in that chapter, if the child or adolescent meets the criteria for any other disorder not mentioned in that section, the other disorder should be diagnosed. For example, the authors indicate that there is no section in this particular chapter on mood disorders and schizophrenia, because the symptoms of these disorders are the same for children, adolescents, and adults. They also suggest that organic mental disorders, psychoactive substance use disorders, schizophreniform disorder, somatoform disorders, sexual disorders, adjustment disorders, and psychological factors affecting physical condition might also be appropriate diagnostic categories for children and adolescents. Personality disorders are included in this list, as well, with some qualifying diagnostic considerations (see the *DSM-III-R*, pp. 335-336). For example, antisocial personality disorder is not diagnosed in children or adolescents until the preceding conduct disorder diagnosis continues after the age of 18 and is pervasive enough to fulfill the criteria for antisocial personality disorder. Conduct disorder, however, may be diagnosed for adults who do not meet the complete criteria for antisocial personality disorder. Avoidant personality disorder and borderline personality disorder (rather than the corresponding categories in the chapter on childhood and adolescence, that is, avoidant disorder of childhood or adolescence or identity disorder, respectively) are diagnosed when the disturbance appears to be pervasive and persistent, and is unlikely to remit as a developmental stage. Additional personality diagnoses may be made with children and adolescents, if the clinician feels the child or adolescent presents unusual personality traits that appear to be consistently maladaptive and likely to be stable over time. A caution is made, however, that the younger the child, the less likelihood there is going to be of "certainty" that the personality disorder will continue indefinitely.

Although not specifically mentioned in the *DSM-III-R's* list of additional disorders the clinician might need to survey in order to diagnose children or adolescents accurately, the section on brief reactive psychosis (pp. 205-207) indicates that the disorder usually appears in adolescence or early adulthood and may need to be considered if the child or adolescent does not meet the diagnostic criteria for other psychotic disorders, especially when there has been a severe stressor that would be upsetting to almost anyone.

Also not mentioned in the list of additional diagnostic categories that might be considered in children and adolescents are the anxiety disorders (or anxiety and phobic neuroses). The *DSM-III-R* mentions that separation anxiety disorder in childhood may predispose the child to develop panic disorder in adulthood (mentioning the age of onset of panic disorder as usually in the late 20s). Likewise, specific mention is made in the chapter on anxiety disorders of the onset of social phobia, usually beginning in late childhood or early adolescence with a typical chronic course that may be exacerbated if anxiety interferes with performance in feared situations. Simple phobia is also mentioned in that animal phobias generally appear in childhood and other specific phobias may begin in adolescence as well. Obsessive-compulsive disorder (or obsessive-compulsive neurosis) is also not mentioned in this list, but onset is thought usually to begin in adolescence or early adulthood and may begin in childhood.

Post-traumatic stress disorder is also not mentioned in this list of possibilities to investigate, but the diagnostic criteria have several references specifically to children and were not included in the *DSM-III* criteria in 1980. Specific mention is made that this disorder can occur at any age (including childhood). However, the *DSM-III-R* still contains rudiments of confusion in diagnosing PTSD in children, stating that children who have been abused (psychologically, physically, or sexually) may evidence a variety of reactions (p. 28). The manual recommends that additional diagnoses constituting a mental disorder be considered in stress-related instances: (a) reactive attachment disorder of infancy or early childhood, (b) post-traumatic stress disorder "(generally for the older child)" (p. 28); and (c) adjustment disorder. Since the age of onset in the anxiety disorder category of PTSD indicates that it can occur at any time (including childhood), it is unclear why the above qualifier implies that it may be more likely to occur in "older" children.

Multiple personality disorder is included in the chapter on dissociative disorders and might need to be considered in children since onset is now thought to be in childhood and predisposing factors have been demonstrated (in almost every case) to have been preceded by abuse or other forms of severe trauma. Evidently this disorder is difficult to diagnose in children as it is typically not identified until the individual is much older. Psychogenic amnesia is also mentioned, which may be coincident with the PTSD diagnosis and is thought to be most often seen in adolescent and young adult females. The amnesia in these cases appears suddenly and is coincident with and a response to the aftermath of a severe psychosocial stress, particularly those stresses involving the threat of physical injury or death, but that type of stress is not required. In addition, depersonalization disorder (or depersonalization neurosis) is thought to be a disorder that occurs in adolescence or adult life and may be a disorder to which a person can be predisposed because of severe stress. The *DSM-III-R* mentions military combat or an automobile accident as examples of factors predisposing to depersonalization disorder. An additional category that might be considered by the clinician is dissociative disorder not otherwise specified.

Sleep disorders may occur, including dyssomnias (i.e., insomnia that can begin at any age, and hypersomnia, which can be related to atypical forms of major depression and is usually "apparent by the 20s," p. 303). Other sleep disorders that might be assessed in children or adolescents who demonstrate sleep disturbances of a severe enough type are sleep-wake schedule disorders (these can occur in the presence of erratic or chaotic conditions and at any age). Dream anxiety disorder (nightmare disorder) is also mentioned as a disorder in which over 50% of the cases begin before the age of 10 and in approximately 66% before the age of 20. The *DSM-III-R* indicates that "a major stressful life event seems to precede the onset of the disorder in about 60% of the cases" (p. 309). Sleep terror disorder also is a disorder that usually begins in childhood (between the ages of 4 and 12) and is often preceded by fatigue or stress.

It is clear that the clinician, in order to be informed about the possibilities of additional stress-related diagnoses, needs to be familiar with all of the categories in the *DSM-III-R* as far as children are concerned. The additional disorders specifically mentioned above have been included because they are diagnoses that can occur in response to stress as a predisposing factor, although stress is not required for many of these diagnoses to be made.

Specific diagnoses mentioned in the *DSM-III-R* chapter on "Disorders Usually First Evident in Infancy, Childhood, or Adolescence" that can be associated with stress, abuse, chaotic circumstances, and so on, are disruptive behavior disorders (including attention-deficit hyperactivity disorder and conduct disorders); anxiety disorders of childhood or adolescence (including separation anxiety disorder); eating disorders (including anorexia nervosa); elimination disorders (including functional encopresis and functional enuresis); and other disorders of infancy, childhood, or adolescence (including elective mutism).

DIFFERENTIAL DIAGNOSES IN ADULTHOOD

For adults, stress-related disorders may include schizophrenia, delusional disorder, brief reactive psychosis, schizophreniform disorder, mood disorders, anxiety disorders, somatoform disorders, adjustment disorders, conversion disorders, hypochondriasis, psychological factors affecting physical condition, dissociative disorders (specifically multiple personality disorder, psychogenic fugue, depersonalization disorder, dissociative disorder not otherwise specified), and sleep disorders (specifically, primary insomnia, primary hypersomnia, dream anxiety disorder, sleep terror disorder, sleepwalking disorder). Organic mental disorders and substance abuse disorders should also be assessed. Personality disorders that may need to be evaluated are antisocial personality disorder (conduct disorder, if full criteria for antisocial personality disorder are not met), paranoid personality disorder, schizotypal personality disorder, borderline personality disorder, and histrionic personality disorder. These personality disorders may predispose the individual to maladaptive responses to stress and may also be interrelated with stress per se (e.g., incest preceding the development of a borderline personality disorder; Stone, 1986, p. 210).

Table 2.1 (pp. 32-39) outlines the possible stress-related disorders, including typical age of onset, predisposing or associated factors (if mentioned in *DSM-III-R* as being stress related), and other factors, which may be considerations but may not be required in making the diagnosis, that might be helpful to the clinician.

GRIEF AND BEREAVEMENT AS POSSIBLE COMPLICATIONS OF STRESS-RELATED DISORDERS

Although several of the stress-related disorders mentioned in the *DSM-III-R* refer to losses involving warfare, combat, and accidents (which generally assume the likelihood of deaths of friends, relatives, or comrades), the only *DSM-III-R*-provided code for a grief or bereavement reaction to these types of losses that do not fulfill other diagnostic criteria is a V Code of uncomplicated bereavement. The V Codes are considered not to be attributable to a "mental disorder," according to the *DSM-III-R*. If individuals do not meet the diagnostic criteria listed in the *DSM-III-R* for any of the other mental disorders, there appears to be no intermediate set of diagnoses for those who suffer a severe reaction to a loss outside of the possibility of disorders not otherwise specified (NOS) included at the end of several of the chapters. These NOS disorders were classified as "atypical" forms of the diagnostic categories in the *DSM-III*. Therefore, outside of the NOS diagnostic possibilities, there may exist a potential void in diagnosing untoward reactions to death or loss of a friend, comrade, or relative between the preceding diagnoses and the V Code of uncomplicated bereavement listed in the *DSM-III-R*.

Garb and his associates (1987) have indicated that there has been an interest in loss and bereavement since Biblical times, but that until the last 40 years it has not captured medical or clinical attention. Although citing military experiences that make it more likely that unresolved grief reactions might occur, they also indicate that research needs to be conducted on this war-traumatized sector that represents, to them, a "somewhat neglected group" (p. 434). They cite, with a case-study example of each, several other possibilities. Those they mention, in addition to what they label "normal grief," include "Absent, Delayed, or Inhibited Grief" (pp. 430-431); "Bereavement Overload" (pp. 431-434); "Chronic Grief" (p. 434); and "Distorted Grief" (pp. 432-433). Grief reactions, in general, can certainly affect individuals to the point of the development of a mental disorder and may be part of the diagnostic syndrome they are experiencing. One of these grief reactions may also exist coincidentally with another mental disorder, as noted by Garb et al. (1987). Haley (1985) indicated that in her work in combat psychiatry, problems often started with the death of a close friend. Although Garb and colleagues are also primarily discussing a military population, it is probable that the diagnostic classification system at our disposal has not identified or diagnosed a portion of the population who may suffer extreme or isolated grief reactions

TABLE 2.1: STRESS-RELATED DISORDERS: COMPOUNDING, CONTRIBUTING, CAUSAL, ASSOCIATED, OR PREDISPOSING FACTORS*

DISORDER	USUAL AGE(S) OF OCCURRENCE	COMPOUNDING, CONTRIBUTING, CAUSAL, ASSOCIATED, OR PREDISPOSING FACTORS
	Disorders Usually Evident in Infancy, Childhood, or Adolescence	
Disruptive Behavior Disorders		
Attention-Deficit Hyperactivity Disorder	Infancy, childhood, adolescence	1. Environmental: chaotic or disorganized 2. Child abuse
Conduct Disorder	Infancy, childhood, adolescence, adulthood	1. Anxiety or depression (may warrant additional diagnoses) 2. Prior attention-deficit hyperactivity disorder or oppositional defiant disorder 3. Rejection - parental or other 4. Discipline and training - harsh or inconsistent 5. Institutionalization - early age 6. Frequent change of residence and caregivers 7. Absence of parent 8. Parent with alcohol dependence 9. Large family 10. Association with delinquent peers

Anxiety Disorders

| Separation Anxiety Disorder | Infancy, childhood, adolescence | 1. Life stress:
a. Loss
b. Death (such as of a relative or a pet)
c. Illness
d. Illness in relative
e. Environmental change |

Eating Disorders

| Anorexia Nervosa | Early - late adolescence to early 30s (late onset is rare) | 1. Stressful life circumstance |

Elimination Disorders

| Functional Encopresis | Infancy, childhood, adolescence | 1. Toilet training: inadequate or inconsistent
2. Psychosocial stress (examples: entry in school, birth of a sibling) |

| Functional Enuresis | Infancy, childhood, adolescence | 1. Psychosocial stress (examples: early hospitalization - between 2 and 4 years of age; entering school, birth of a sibling) |

Other Disorders

| Elective Mutism | Infancy, childhood, adolescence | 1. Overprotection by parent
2. Having language or speech disorders, or mental retardation
3. Immigration
4. Hospitalization or trauma before 3 years of age |

33

DISORDER	USUAL AGE(S) OF OCCURRENCE	COMPOUNDING, CONTRIBUTING, CAUSAL, ASSOCIATED, OR PREDISPOSING FACTORS
	Schizophrenia	
Schizophrenia	Any age: Usually begins in adolescence or early adulthood. May begin in middle or late adult life	1. Onset or exacerbation may occur as a result of a psychosocial stressor
	Delusional (Paranoid) Disorder	
Delusional Disorder	Generally in middle or late adult life, but can begin at younger ages. Average age: 40-55	1. Immigration or emigration 2. Being deaf 3. Severe stresses
	Psychotic Disorders Not Classified Elsewhere	
Brief Reactive Psychosis	Adolescence or early adulthood	1. Event(s) that when taken alone or in combination with each other would be extremely stressful to almost anyone experiencing those stressor(s). Examples: loss of someone one loves; combat 2. Diagnoses of schizophrenia or schizotypal personality disorder supersede this diagnosis 3. A psychotic mood disorder or factors of organic origin also supersede this diagnosis

4. Pre-existing psychopathology may render a person vulnerable to this disorder
5. Pre-existing personality disorders may also make a person vulnerable to this disorder. Both diagnoses may be made
6. Pre-existing major stress is <u>required</u> for diagnosis of this disorder
7. Manic or major depressive disorders supersede this diagnosis, <u>regardless</u> of whether the person has experienced a major psychosocial stressor

Schizophreniform Disorder

1. In situations where criteria are met for <u>both</u> brief reactive psychosis and schizophreniform disorder, brief reactive psychosis preempts that of schizophreniform disorder if (a) the symptoms last only 3-4 weeks and (b) the symptoms do not meet the criteria required for a diagnosis of schizophrenia

Mood Disorders

Manic Episode

Average age of onset is in the early 20s but a large number of new cases appear after age 50

1. Psychosocial stressors
2. Antidepressants (either medication or electroconvulsive therapy [ECT])
3. Childbirth

Major Depressive Episode

Average age is in the late 20s, but can begin at any age <u>including infancy</u>

1. May develop over days or weeks (or suddenly) especially when coping with severe psychosocial stress
2. Physical disorders

DISORDER	USUAL AGE(S) OF OCCURRENCE	COMPOUNDING, CONTRIBUTING, CAUSAL, ASSOCIATED, OR PREDISPOSING FACTORS
Mood Disorders (Continued)		
Dysthymia	Childhood, adolescence, or early adult life	1. Physical illness or conditions 2. Chronic psychosocial stressors
	Children or adolescents	1. Attention-deficit hyperactivity disorder, conduct disorder, mental retardation, or a severe specific developmental disorder predispose an individual to dysthymia 2. Environment: inadequate, rejecting, disorganized, or chaotic 3. Common in those with personality disorders: histrionic, narcissistic, avoidant, or dependent
Anxiety Disorders		
Panic Disorder	Onset: average age is late 20s	1. Separation anxiety disorder in childhood 2. Loss of social support system(s) 3. Disrupted interpersonal relationships that are important to the individual
Post-Traumatic Stress Disorder	Any age, including childhood	1. Pre-existing psychopathological conditions predispose the individual to PTSD 2. Can develop in individuals without pre-existing disorders, especially if the stressor is of great magnitude

3. Extreme stressor(s) - upsetting to almost anyone - <u>is required</u> for this diagnosis

Somatoform Disorders

Conversion Disorder	Adolescence or early adulthood. Middle age or later	1. Extreme psychological or psychosocial stress. Examples: warfare; death of a significant person 2. Physical disorders 3. Exposure to people with physical disorders or conversion symptoms 4. Personality disorders predispose to this disorder (histrionic or dependent personality disorders)
Hypochondriasis	Any age. Average onset: 20-30	1. Organic disease 2. Organic disease of family member or other significant figure 3. Psychosocial stressor(s)
Somatoform Pain Disorder	Any age, including childhood. Average onset: 30s and 40s	1. In 50% the pain starts after a physical trauma

Dissociative Disorders

Multiple Personality Disorder	Invariably in childhood - it is usually not diagnosed until much later	1. Abuse: physical or sexual 2. Severe emotional trauma in childhood

DISORDER	USUAL AGE(S) OF OCCURRENCE	COMPOUNDING, CONTRIBUTING, CAUSAL, ASSOCIATED, OR PREDISPOSING FACTORS
	Dissociative Disorders (Continued)	
Psychogenic Fugue	Varies	1. Heavy use of alcohol 2. Typically follows severe psychosocial stress. Examples: marital fights, rejections, military activities (such as in wartime), or natural disasters
Psychogenic Amnesia	Usually in adolescents and females in early adulthood. Young males in the military during wartime	1. Sudden amnesia following severe psychosocial stress 2. Stressors involving threats of injury or death
Depersonalization Disorder	Adolescents/young adults	1. Severe stress. Examples: combat, auto accidents
Dissociative Disorder Not Otherwise Specified	Any age (?) Children	1. In children, this disorder may develop following physical abuse or trauma 2. Periods of extensive coercive persuasion (i.e., activities perpetrated by terrorists or cultists while being held captive)
	Sleep Disorders	
Dyssomnias		
Insomnia Disorders	Any age, but may be exacerbated or become more common with aging	1. Psychosocial stressor(s) 2. More common in individuals with higher levels of stress or psychopathology

Parasomnias

Disorder	Onset	Features
Dream Anxiety Disorder (Nightmare Disorder)	Onset: 50% begin before 10 years of age, 66% before 20	1. Increase in mental stress 2. Physical fatigue 3. Changes in the individual's sleeping environment 4. 60% have major stress prior to development of this disorder
Sleep Terror Disorder	Onset: children - usually 4-12 years of age, adults - 20s or 30s	1. Fatigue 2. Stress
Sleepwalking Disorder	Onset: usually 6-12 years of age	1. Fatigue 2. Stress

Adjustment Disorders

Disorder	Onset	Features
Adjustment Disorders	Any age	1. Single, multiple, recurrent, or continuous stressors 2. Chronic illness 3. Natural disasters 4. Persecution 5. Vulnerable individuals may have a more extreme reaction to stressors

*Source: American Psychiatric Association. (1987). Diagnostic and Statistical Manual of Mental Disorders (3rd ed. rev.). Washington, DC: Author. Copyright © by the American Psychiatric Association. Adapted with permission.

that might not be identified by our existing mental-disorder classification or occur in conjunction with another mental disorder.

An additional point often noted by those suffering from PTSD is an inability to talk about stressful losses, psychic numbing, and so on. The possibility exists that this is a cultural phenomenon in that talking about losses is not encouraged, and may even be actively discouraged. Such statements as "Get on with it!" and "Haven't you cried enough?" are indications that people, in general, do not want to hear about these vulnerabilities. The more profound the loss, the greater is the tendency to discourage active mourning. Perhaps, in addition, the greater the pain, the greater is the inability to discuss it - the greater is the embarrassment. These factors may also contribute to the "neglected group" cited by Garb and his associates (1987).

DIFFERENTIAL DIAGNOSIS AND COMPOUNDING DISORDERS THAT MAY NOT BE REACTIONS TO SPECIFIC OR IDENTIFIED SEVERE STRESSORS

Some diagnoses may or may not be related to specific or severe stressors. These may include somatization disorder, factitious disorder, substance abuse disorders, antisocial personality disorder, and malingering.

The assessment of somatization disorder needs to include previous medical and psychological history because this disorder begins early in one's development (rarely as late as the 20s - American Psychiatric Association, 1987). Because of its early development, it is more likely to have been present prior to a stressor. This disorder was once called hysteria and has also been referred to as Briquet's syndrome (Goodwin & Guze, 1984). The hallmark of somatization disorder (American Psychiatric Association, 1987) is many somatic problems that are continually presented to physicians over the course of many years. Furthermore, the symptoms often form a vague pattern and are presented in equally vague or dramatic ways. The configurations of complaints are such that no apparent actual physical disorder can be documented or diagnosed to explain the symptoms presented. This disorder persists and waxes and wanes for years (American Psychiatric Association, 1987). According to the *DSM-III-R*, "antisocial behavior and occupational, interpersonal, and marital difficulties are common" (p. 262). Goodwin and Guze (1984) also discuss antisocial personality difficulties in both males and females in addressing complications involving somatization disorder.

The person with somatization disorder, therefore, has a history of many medical consultations, tests, and evaluations; hospitalizations; many unnecessary surgeries; or all of these. Substance use abuse is a common problem, especially when related to the use of a number of prescription medications. Substance abuse can lead to completed suicides.

The *DSM-III-R* indicates that physical disorders that also involve "vague, multiple, and confusing symptoms [e.g., hyperparathyroidism, porphyria, multiple sclerosis, and systemic lupus erythematosus]" (American Psychiatric Association, 1987, p. 263) must be ruled out. A major problem with somatization disorder is that an actual organic disease can be missed, which accounts for the continual searching for such a disease. The hazards of such continuous "searching" have already been mentioned in terms of the complications inherent with surgery, in general, and in the compounding of iatrogenic problems with multiple medications and the interactions among them that can produce physical and mental symptoms of their own. Somatization disorder with onset in older individuals presenting many physical complaints almost *invariably* indicates that a true physical disorder is present (American Psychiatric Association, 1987).

Factitious disorders, in which the individual apparently has voluntary control over the presentation of symptoms, needs to be examined also. The person presents symptoms in this disorder that do not fit a picture of other mental disorders. This person needs to be in the patient role, "needs to be sick," and, therefore, the fact of previous hospitalizations must be established. Like somatization disorder, the factitious disorder is likely to have been present prior to a traumatic stressor. Individuals who fit the *DSM-III-R* criteria for factitious disorder may also have evidenced one or more of the personality disorders (listed in the *DSM-III-R*). Therefore, it is generally important to review those criteria to ascertain whether the individual fits into any of the personality disorder categories.

Some have suggested that alcohol or other substance abuse must be ruled out before a diagnosis of PTSD can be unconditionally made. Jelinek and Williams (1984) have indicated that substance abuse can (a) suppress, (b) exacerbate, or (c) perpetuate the symptoms of PTSD. Therefore, the use or possible abuse of any substance needs to be assessed. These authors suggest that the clinician differentiate among those with PTSD who are (a) without alcohol abuse, (b) with alcohol abuse, and (c) with lifelong histories of alcohol abuse. Others have also suggested that the assessment should inquire into whether any alcohol abuse or abuse of other substances occurred or increased after the trauma, because these abuses may also be evidence that the individual has been trying to self-medicate (Blank, 1985; Brett & Ostroff, 1985, citing Kardiner & Spiegel; Burgess & Holmstrom, 1974; Lipkin et al., 1985). This effort to self-medicate one's psychological or physical symptoms may be an effort to calm down, go to sleep, or dull oneself against daytime memories or nightmares. Therefore, it is important to ascertain whether substance abuse became worse or started after the trauma for it to have diagnostic significance. However, alcohol or other substance abuse and withdrawal have their own sets of symptoms and are not the only symptoms caused by a significant stressor outside the realm of normal experience. The *DSM-III-R* indicates that assessment for substance use disorders and organic mental disorders be routinely made in assessing any disorder. The *DSM-III-R* indicates that if an organic mental disorder develops after the trauma, this additional diagnosis may be given. Caffeine intake can also contribute to anxiety, and the investigator should inquire about its use (Ziskin, 1981a).

Although many individuals with PTSD fulfill some of the *DSM-III-R* criteria for antisocial personality disorder (Brett & Ostroff, 1985, citing Walker), this disorder is of long standing. Individuals with personality disorders generally evidence them by the time they reach their mid-teenage years. Therefore, even though people with PTSD also have some of the antisocial personality disorder characteristics, it is important to assess the existence of this personality disorder by evaluating symptoms appearing before the age of 15. Aspects of the personality disorder that appear *only after* the existence of an extreme stressor are, therefore, more likely to have been caused by the stressor and not by an antisocial personality disorder. It is likely that individuals with an antisocial personality disorder are no more immune to severe stressors than anyone else (and may even be more vulnerable to them);

however, one is reminded of the little boy who cried, "Wolf." Existence of this personality disorder makes it less likely that judges and juries will believe that the production of symptoms of PTSD have not been manufactured.

Bailey (1985) indicated that comparing individuals with PTSD and those with antisocial personality disorder was difficult because of some of the similarities found in both (hostility, aggressivity, tendency to blame others, suspiciousness - particularly of authority figures, and problems in relationships with others). However, he recommended that the social history of the individual might provide differentiating information. In addition to pretrauma antisocial difficulties not evident in those with PTSD, persons with PTSD may be more likely to express feelings of guilt and have difficulties with disparities in value systems (i.e., pretrauma behavior and behavior engaged in for survival purposes) than persons with antisocial personality disorder. Since a complication in this differential is the "emotional numbing" that many survivors experience, this may not be a helpful discrimination in many cases. This leaves, once again, a previous history with evidence of antisocial personality disorder as the discriminant. Sparr and Atkinson (1986) and Hoffman (1986) also stressed prior history of delinquency as an especially helpful differentiating factor. In addition, Hoffman emphasized that the clinician must be alert to observations regarding the patient's honesty. He suggested that a history of previous "accidents" and resulting "lawsuits" might also be differentiating factors, and thus, the clinician must make inquiries about these aspects of a patient's history. This latter differential might also be useful in the determination of malingering.

The last area to be examined is suspicion of malingering. It is indeed unfortunate that the *DSM-III* did not establish extensive criteria for the malingering aspect of assessment. One seems always to be confronted with the question: "Is this person faking symptoms to achieve monetary or secondary gains?" It is even more discouraging to find that in the *DSM-III-R* the criteria remained the same. Obviously, further study is necessary in this area.

A person requires two or more of the following to qualify for suspicion of malingering. It is important to note that the *DSM-III* did not actually have a diagnostic category for malingering; the four criteria mentioned only served to "cast suspicion." Two of the following four, therefore, needed to be present: (a) the person is referred by his or her attorney in a legal context to a physician or a psychologist; (b) there is a discernible gap between the person's claimed level of distress "or disability and the objective findings" (p. 360); (c) the person does not cooperate fully with the diagnostic evaluation, assessment, and prescriptions for treatment; and (d) the person evidences "the presence of Antisocial Personality Disorder" (p. 360).

There are problems with the first three criteria involved in the suspicion of malingering category. First, it is possible that a person might be referred for medical or psychological evaluation by an attorney who is concerned that the person might be reacting to extreme stress or have a psychological disorder. Just as friends, relatives, or employers might be the first people in one's environment to notice distress, attorneys may notice it as well (Modlin, 1967). It has been evident that individuals who experience distress seek various avenues to relieve it, among them the legal avenue. Researchers involved in the Buffalo Creek disaster, for example, found that when this community became involved in litigation against the mining company for reckless negligence, its members seemed to pull together and to deal with their psychological symptoms better (Wilkinson & Vera, 1985).

Second, the evaluator notices that there is a discrepancy between the individual's claims of distress and the available or actual evidence. It has already been mentioned that individuals' responses to stressors vary considerably. People can develop a number of psychological disorders following an extreme stressor. In addition, researchers have indicated that individuals with PTSD may attempt to minimize their symptoms and may not wish to discuss them fully because of guilt, lack of trust, and so on. Individuals are often "embarrassed" by their psychological symptoms. Other people do not understand the symptoms and may see the person as "peculiar."

Some people present symptoms of distress as pleas for assistance. If they find the symptoms already intolerable, and if other people have not understood them, how do they get the attention they need to obtain help in alleviating their distress? It is not uncommon for people suffering from extreme stress to become demanding and appear to exaggerate to make their distress clearer to those around them. It is like trying to communicate to someone who does not speak English. Everyone knows that if you speak more slowly or "yell," the person will be "more likely to understand you."

The third *DSM-III-R* criterion for suspicion of malingering is that the person does not cooperate with the diagnostic evaluation and prescriptions for treatment. It has already been mentioned that individuals with PTSD may drop out of therapy and may refuse to continue prescribed treatment (Burstein, 1986; Fox & Scherl, 1972; Jackson et al., 1985). Guilt (Lifton, 1982; Lindy, 1985; Smith, 1982; West & Coburn, 1984), distrust in the solidity and safety of the environment (Arthur & McKenna, 1983; Garb et al., 1987; Lifton, 1982; Lindy, 1985; McKenna & Arthur, 1983), and recurrent associations with the trauma by talking about it may be psychically and emotionally painful (Boehnlein et al., 1985; Lindy, 1985); talking about it also may add more associations to the others already related to the trauma. There is a sincere desire to "forget" and to "remove oneself" as mentioned in the "psychic numbing" subcategory of the *DSM-III-R* (Burgess & Holmstrom, 1974; Cornfield & Hogben, 1980; Jackson et al., 1985; Kinzie et al., 1984; Wilkinson, 1985). All of these factors that are experienced by individuals with PTSD are factors that enter into the *DSM-III-R* criteria of suspicion of malingering.

Evidence of an antisocial personality disorder, therefore, is about what is left unsullied by a PTSD individual's reactions to an extreme stressor. Antisocial personality disorder has its roots in the individual's development before the age of 15, and the investigation of malingering should start there.

Was the child or adolescent (before the age of 15) truant (often)? Did he or she run away from home more than once or not return home at least once? Did the juvenile start physical fights, use a weapon more than once during such fights, or force someone into a sexual encounter? Was the individual physically cruel to animals or other people? Did he or she destroy other people's property, set fires, or tell lies other than those that were told in an effort to avoid physical or sexual abuse from another? Did the individual steal with or without confrontation with the victim? Three or more of these 12 items are required prior to the age of 15 before the diagnosis of antisocial personality disorder can be established. By definition, personality disorders are of long duration. Of course, in order to warrant the diagnosis, the individual must also meet the rest of the criteria in the

45

DSM-III-R after the age of 15 and well into adult life, but if what we are confronted with is ascertaining pre-stress and post-stress related behaviors, these prior behaviors must be taken into account. This is also true of somatization disorder and factitious disorder. Malingering includes the possibility that the person with an antisocial personality disorder is deliberately attempting to obtain some sort of personal gain (monetary or otherwise) and is not, therefore, likely to be suffering inordinately from a stress-related mental disorder. Likewise, the possibility of the existence of an antisocial personality disorder as an associated feature and as a familial pattern in an individual with somatization disorder must also alert the clinician to the possibility that monetary or other gain could be related to the presentation of symptoms (i.e., as seen in unwarranted disability claims). Table 2.2 (pp. 47-49) presents information regarding age-related factors and other data that might be important in assessment.

Obviously, information in this area is difficult to obtain and it is a portion of the field of psychological research that may be determined solely by litigation and forensic legal practice.

TESTING

Ziskin (1981a, 1981b, 1981c) suggests that if the evaluator has not administered the Minnesota Multiphasic Personality Inventory (MMPI), the attorney for the defense should ask for one. Research on assessment of stress-related disorders with the MMPI is relatively new and tentative. However, the utilization of the validity scales may be useful to the court. What was the person's test-taking attitude? Did he or she try to fake good or bad, gloss over symptoms, or exaggerate them? Did the person answer the questions honestly? This information may be of value to the court regarding the "character" and "personality structure" of the individual. The testing is unlikely to elicit answers to questions regarding the significance and nature of an extreme stressor. It is not going to provide differential diagnostic classification of the stress-related disorders mentioned. It may give an indication, however, of how depressed or anxious the person is, about how much he or she is dwelling on physiological and other symptoms, and the presence of an antiso-

TABLE 2.2: DISORDERS THAT MAY NOT BE DUE TO REACTIONS TO SPECIFIC OR EXTREME STRESSORS*

DISORDER	USUAL AGE(S) OF OCCURRENCE	COMPOUNDING, CONTRIBUTING, CAUSAL, ASSOCIATED, OR PREDISPOSING FACTORS
Factitious Disorders		
Factitious Disorders with Physical Symptoms	Usually, onset is in young adulthood	1. Needs to be in a "sick" or patient role 2. May begin with hospitalization for an actual physical illness 3. Lifelong series of hospitalizations 4. Dramatic description of symptoms 5. Disrupts hospital routines, argues, or refuses to follow hospital regulations 6. Extremely knowledgeable about medical terms and hospital procedures 7. Continued use of pain medications 8. Previous surgeries 9. When physical disorders are not located, new symptoms are produced 10. No external incentives for this disorder are present
Factitious Disorder with Psychological Symptoms	DSM-III-R includes no information	1. Severe personality disorder is invariably present 2. Needs to be in a sick or patient role 3. Symptoms "worse" when the person is obviously being observed 4. Suggestible: Complains of symptoms mentioned earlier by others

DISORDER	USUAL AGE(S) OF OCCURRENCE	COMPOUNDING, CONTRIBUTING, CAUSAL, ASSOCIATED, OR PREDISPOSING FACTORS
		Factitious Disorders (Continued)
		5. Negative or uncooperative
		6. Symptoms not confirmed by others who are in a position to observe them
		7. Use of substances to produce "intended" symptoms
		8. No external incentives for this disorder are present
		Somatoform Disorder
Somatization Disorder	Before age 30 and lasting several years. Onset: teenage years or in the person's 20s	1. Continuing multiple physical complaints over many years
		2. No physical disorder found that would explain the symptoms or would be significant enough for the extensiveness of the symptoms
		3. Complaints that are vague, dramatic, exaggerated, or have a complex medical history
		4. Anxiety or depression may exist
		5. Disturbed interpersonal relationships and chaotic lifestyle
		6. Personality disorders: histrionic or antisocial personality disorder
		7. Psychoactive substance abuse or resultant suicide

8. Relatives (both biological and adoptive) of people with this disorder have a higher incidence of somatic, psychoactive substance use disorders, or antisocial personality disorders

9. Onset of many symptoms late in life (DSM-III-R, p. 263) is almost always due to physical disease

Malingering

Malingering	No information

1. Symptom production is due to external incentive(s)
2. Legal or medical context
3. Unable to confirm individual's claim(s) of stress or disability
4. Antisocial personality disorder

Antisocial Personality Disorder

Antisocial Personality Disorder	18 years old or older

1. Conduct Disorder before 15 years of age

*Source: American Psychiatric Association. (1987). Diagnostic and Statistical Manual of Mental Disorders (3rd ed. rev.). Washington, DC: Author. Copyright © by the American Psychiatric Association. Adapted with permission.

49

cial personality disorder. How much these personality or attitudinal factors have been compounded as a result of the stressors is still likely to be open to conjecture.

It is generally not helpful to send individuals with psychological impairments to many different evaluators because that, alone, tends to exacerbate distress and concern about their functioning, future, and prognosis. However, it has been apparent that it is important to remove testing evaluations from the aforementioned history taking and therapy involvement to another therapist for this aspect of assessment. If the test is conducted by the same person doing the previously mentioned evaluation, and if what is required by "testing" is the desire for even greater "evidence of objectivity," then this is a factor that needs to be considered.

If the interpreter of the test data and the therapist independently substantiate conclusions regarding the evaluation and assessment of the existence of a disorder, this adds more diagnostic credibility to the process. It behooves attorneys, therefore, to seek a qualified therapist and a qualified interpreter of psychological scales and to work with them individually, with no conjoint consultation between the psychological specialists.

Some research evidence has been cited to demonstrate that preliminary studies indicate some scale differences on the MMPI or other tests among those who have PTSD, those who have not been adjudged (by experts) to have it (Arnold, 1985, citing research by others; Bailey, 1985; Fairbank, McCaffrey, & Keane, 1985), and those who are faking good or bad after having been coached on the *DSM-III* criteria of PTSD (Fairbank et al., 1985). Fairbank and associates achieved a 90% detection rate after fabricators were coached by experts to simulate the symptoms of PTSD. They were compared with 15 veterans who had been diagnosed as actually having the disorder. The actual PTSD subjects were determined, however, utilizing the *DSM-III* criteria; history and additional assessment procedures (not specified) were developed by the authors.

SELF-EVALUATION OF
DIFFICULTIES QUESTIONNAIRE

The Self-Evaluation of Difficulties Questionnaire (see Appendix, pp. 195-215) may help the examiner to order events chronologically in the person's life and to acquaint himself or herself with previous difficulties that may have predisposed the individual to gross stress reactions to an extreme stressor. The self-evaluation may also give the examiner some clues regarding other areas that need to be explored, since some individuals may find it easier to write down their thoughts and feelings than to discuss them with a stranger.

The self-evaluation questionnaire also helps the clinician to outline many areas of difficulties likely to be experienced by individuals suffering from stress-related disorders. Since, as has already been noted, people often find it difficult to discuss their problems with another person, the fact that this task is presented as a self-evaluation helps people feel that they have a greater role and more control in the process. Also, completeness is emphasized and the categories help them recall difficulties they may have forgotten to discuss with the therapist. Once written, the information seems to be easier to talk about and the therapist can make further inquiries in a sensitive manner. Since people complete this task on their own and bring it into therapy at a later time, it seems to be less threatening. The person feels less "scrutinized" or "on the spot." Some individuals have even stated that they felt it was therapeutic just to complete this project.

It is hoped that research in this and related areas will continue. The carefulness and specificity of the *DSM-III*, and, now, the *DSM-III-R's* diagnostic criteria, greatly advanced understanding regarding the nature of disorders, and how they are ultimately differentiated from one another.

Carroll L. Meek, PhD, has been in independent practice as a counseling psychologist since 1982. For 13 years prior to this, she was in Counseling Services at Washington State University, Pullman. She received her BA degree in psychology from Whitman College, Walla Walla, WA in 1964; her MS degree in student personnel in higher education from Indiana University, Bloomington, IN in 1966; and her PhD degree in guidance and counseling from the University of Idaho, Moscow, ID in 1972. In addition to her work at Washington State University, she was a counselor at the University of Idaho's Counseling Center for 1 year and was a counselor and head resident at the University of Wisconsin, Oshkosh, for 2 years. Dr. Meek may be contacted at The Professional Mall, S.E. 1205 Professional Mall Boulevard, Pullman, WA 99163.

REFERENCES

Allen, I. M. (1986, January). Posttraumatic stress disorder among Black Vietnam veterans. *Hospital and Community Psychiatry, 37,* 55-61.

American Psychiatric Association. (1980). *Diagnostic and Statistical Manual of Mental Disorders* (3rd ed.). Washington, DC: Author.

American Psychiatric Association. (1987). *Diagnostic and Statistical Manual of Mental Disorders* (3rd ed. rev.). Washington, DC: Author.

Andreasen, N. C. (1980). Posttraumatic stress disorder. In H. I. Kaplan, A. M. Freedman, & B. J. Sadock (Eds.), *Comprehensive Textbook of Psychiatry-III* (Vol. 2, 3rd ed., pp. 1517-1525). Baltimore: Williams & Wilkins.

Archibald, H. C., Long, D. M., Miller, C., & Tuddenham, R. D. (1962, October). Gross stress reaction in combat--A 15-year follow-up. *American Journal of Psychiatry, 119,* 317-322.

Arnold, A. L. (1985). Diagnosis of post-traumatic stress disorder in Viet Nam veterans. In S. M. Sonnenberg, A. S. Blank, & J. A. Talbott (Eds.), *The Trauma of War: Stress and Recovery in Viet Nam Veterans* (pp. 99-124). Washington, DC: American Psychiatric Press.

Arthur, R. J., & McKenna, G. J. (1983). Survival under conditions of extreme stress. *Directions in Psychiatry, 3,* (Lesson 35), 1-7.

Atkinson, R. M., Henderson, R. G., Sparr, L. F., & Deale, S. (1982, September). Assessment of Viet Nam veterans for posttraumatic stress disorder in Veterans Administration disability claims. *American Journal of Psychiatry, 139,* 1118-1121.

Atkinson, R. M., Sparr, L. F., Sheff, A. G., White, R. A. F., & Fitzsimmons, J. T. (1984, May). Diagnosis of post-traumatic stress disorder in Viet Nam veterans: Preliminary findings. *American Journal of Psychiatry, 141,* 694-696.

Bailey, J. E. (1985, August). Differential diagnosis of posttraumatic stress and antisocial personality disorders. *Hospital and Community Psychiatry, 36,* 881-883.

Beigel, A., & Berren, M. R. (1985, March). Human-induced disasters. *Psychiatric Annals, 15,* 143-144, 147-148, 150.

Benedek, E. D. (1985, March). Children and disaster: Emerging issues. *Psychiatric Annals, 15,* 168-172.

Blank, A. S. (1985). Irrational reactions to post-traumatic stress disorder and Viet Nam veterans. In S. M. Sonnenberg, A. S. Blank, & J. A. Talbott (Eds.), *The Trauma of War: Stress and Recovery in Viet Nam Veterans* (pp. 69-98). Washington, DC: American Psychiatric Press.

Bloch, A. M. (1978, October). Combat neurosis in innercity schools. *American Journal of Psychiatry, 135,* 1189-1192.

Boehnlein, J. K., Kinzie, J. D., Ben, R., & Fleck, J. (1985, August). One-year follow-up study of posttraumatic stress disorder among survivors of Cambodian concentration camps. *American Journal of Psychiatry, 142,* 956-959.

Boulanger, G. (1985). Post-traumatic stress disorder: An old problem with a new name. In S. M. Sonnenberg, A. S. Blank, & J. A. Talbott (Eds.), *The Trauma of War: Stress and Recovery in Viet Nam Veterans* (pp. 13-29). Washington, DC: American Psychiatric Press.

Braceland, F. J. (1982, November). Forgotten men. *Psychiatric Annals, 12,* 975-976.

Breslau, N., & Davis, G. C. (1987, May). Posttraumatic stress disorder: The etiologic specificity of wartime stressors. *American Journal of Psychiatry, 144,* 578-583.

Brett, E. A., & Ostroff, R. (1985, April). Imagery and posttraumatic stress disorder: An overview. *American Journal of Psychiatry, 142,* 417-424.

Bromberg, W. (1984a, July). Introduction. *Psychiatric Annals, 11,* 497-498.

Bromberg, W. (1984b, July). Psychiatric traumatology. *Psychiatric Annals, 11,* 500-505.

Burgess, A. W., & Holmstrom, L. L. (1974, September). Rape trauma syndrome. *American Journal of Psychiatry, 131,* 981-986.

Burstein, A. (1986, January). Treatment noncompliance in patients with post-traumatic stress disorder. *Psychosomatics, 27,* 37-40.

Byrne, K. (1985). Conducting the initial forensic interview. In P. A. Keller & L. G. Ritt (Eds.), *Innovations in Clinical Practice: A Source Book* (Vol. 4, pp. 467-474). Sarasota, FL: Professional Resource Exchange.

Christenson, R. M., Walker, J. I., Ross, D. R., & Maltbie, A. A. (1981, July). Reactivation of traumatic conflicts. *American Journal of Psychiatry, 138,* 984-985.

Corcoran, J. F. T. (1982, November). The concentration camp syndrome and USAF Vietnam prisoners of war. *Psychiatric Annals, 12,* 991-994.

Cornfield, R. B., & Hogben, G. (1980). Traumatic neuroses of war. *Weekly Psychiatric Update Series, 3* (Lesson 30). Princeton, NJ: Biomedia.

Dimsdale, J. E. (1974, July). The coping behavior of nazi concentration camp survivors. *American Journal of Psychiatry, 131,* 792-797.

Dunn, C. G. (1981, January). The diagnosis and classification of anxiety states. *Psychiatric Annals, 11,* 11-14, 16.

Eaton, W. W., Sigal, J. J., & Weinfeld, M. (1982, June). Impairment in Holocaust survivors after 33 years: Data from an unbiased community sample. *American Journal of Psychiatry, 139,* 773-777.

Erikson, K. T. (1976, March). Loss of communality at Buffalo Creek. *American Journal of Psychiatry, 133,* 302-305.

Ettedgui, E., & Bridges, M. (1985, March). Posttraumatic stress disorder. *Psychiatric Clinics of North America, 8,* 89-103.

Fairbank, J. A., McCaffrey, R. J., & Keane, T. M. (1985, April). Psychometric detection of fabricated symptoms of posttraumatic stress disorder. *American Journal of Psychiatry, 142,* 501-503.

Faravelli, C., Webb, T., Ambonetti, A., Fonnesu, F., & Sessarego, A. (1985, December). Prevalence of traumatic early life events in 31 agoraphobic patients with panic attacks. *American Journal of Psychiatry, 142,* 1493-1494.

Finkelhor, D. (1987, April). The sexual abuse of children: Current research reviewed. *Psychiatric Annals, 17,* 233-237, 241.

Fox, S. S., & Scherl, D. J. (1972, January). Crisis intervention with victims of rape. *Social Work,* pp. 37-42.

Foy, D. W., Donahoe, C. P., Jr., Carroll, E. M., Gallers, J., & Reno, R. (1987). Posttraumatic stress disorder. In L. Michelson & L. M. Ascher (Eds.), *Anxiety and Stress Disorders: Cognitive-Behavioral Assessment and Treatment* (pp. 361-378). New York: Guilford.

Friedman, M. J., Schneiderman, C. K., West, A. N., & Corson, J. A. (1986, April). Measurement of combat exposure, posttraumatic stress disorder, and life stress among Vietnam combat veterans. *American Journal of Psychiatry, 143,* 537-539.

Frye, J. S., & Stockton, R. A. (1982, January). Discriminant analysis of posttraumatic stress disorder among a group of Viet Nam veterans. *American Journal of Psychiatry, 139,* 52-56.

Garb, R., Bleich, A., & Lerer, B. (1987, September). Bereavement in combat. *The Psychiatric Clinics of North America, 10,* 421-436.

Goodwin, D. W., & Guze, S. B. (1984). Hysteria (somatization disorder). In *Psychiatric Diagnosis* (3rd ed., pp. 89-108). New York: Oxford University Press.

Groesbeck, C. J. (1982, November). Dreams of a Vietnam veteran--A Jungian analytic perspective. *Psychiatric Annals, 12,* 1007-1008, 1010.

Haley, S. A. (1985, Spring). Some of my best friends are dead: Treatment of the post-traumatic stress disorder patient and his family. *Family Systems Medicine, 3,* 17-26.

Hall, R. C. W., & Malone, P. T. (1976, July). Psychiatric effects of prolonged Asian captivity: A two-year follow-up. *American Journal of Psychiatry, 133,* 786-790.

Hamilton, J. D. V., & Canteen, W. (1987, February). Post-traumatic stress disorder in World War II naval veterans. *Hospital and Community Psychiatry, 38,* 197-199.

Hendin, H., Pollinger, A., Singer, P., & Ulman, R. B. (1981, November). Meanings of combat and the development of posttraumatic stress disorder. *American Journal of Psychiatry, 138,* 1490-1493.

Hillman, R. G. (1981, September). The psychopathology of being held hostage. *American Journal of Psychiatry, 138,* 1193-1197.

Hoffman, B. F. (1986, February). How to write a psychiatric report for litigation following a personal injury. *American Journal of Psychiatry, 143,* 164-169.

Hoiberg, A., & McCaughey, B. G. (1984, January). The traumatic aftereffects of collision at sea. *American Journal of Psychiatry, 143,* 70-73.

Horowitz, M. J. (1985, March). Disasters and psychological responses to stress. *Psychiatric Annals, 15,* 161-163, 166-167.

Horowitz, M. J. (1986, March). Stress-response syndromes: A review of posttraumatic and adjustment disorders. *Hospital and Community Psychiatry, 37,* 241-249.

Jackson, T. L., Quevillon, R. P., & Petretic-Jackson, P. A. (1985). Assessment and treatment of sexual assault victims. In P. A. Keller & L. G. Ritt (Eds.), *Innovations in Clinical Practice: A Source Book* (Vol. 4, pp. 51-78). Sarasota, FL: Professional Resource Exchange.

Jelinek, J. M., & Williams, T. (1984). Post-traumatic stress disorder and substance abuse in Vietnam combat veterans: Treatment problems, strategies and recommendations. *Journal of Substance Abuse Treatment, 1,* 87-97.

Kinzie, J. D., Fredrickson, R. H., Ben, R., Fleck, J., & Karls, W. (1984, May). Posttraumatic stress disorder among survivors of Cambodian concentration camps. *American Journal of Psychiatry, 141,* 645-650.

Kolb, L. C., & Mutalipassi, L. R. (1982, November). The conditioned emotional response: A sub-class of the chronic and delayed post-traumatic stress disorder. *Psychiatric Annals, 12,* 979-981, 984-987.

Laufer, R. S., Brett, E., & Gallops, M. S. (1985, November). Symptom patterns associated with posttraumatic stress disorder among Vietnam veterans exposed to war trauma. *American Journal of Psychiatry, 142,* 1304-1311.

Lavie, P., Hefez, A., Halperin, G., & Enoch, D. (1979, February). Long-term effects of traumatic war-related events on sleep. *American Journal of Psychiatry, 136,* 175-178.

Leopold, R. L., & Dillon, H. (1963, April). Psychoanatomy of a disaster: A long term study of post-traumatic neuroses in survivors of a marine explosion. *American Journal of Psychiatry, 119,* 913-921.

Levav, I. L., Greenfeld, H., & Baruch, E. (1979, May). Psychiatric combat reactions during the Yom Kippur War. *American Journal of Psychiatry, 136,* 637-641.

Lifton, R. J. (1982, November). The psychology of the survivor and the death imprint. *Psychiatric Annals, 12,* 1011-1012, 1014-1017, 1020.

Lindberg, F. H., & Distad, L. J. (1985). Post-traumatic stress disorders in women who experienced childhood incest. *Child Abuse & Neglect, 8,* 329-334.

Lindy, J. D. (1985, March). The trauma membrane and other clinical concepts derived from psychotherapeutic work with survivors of natural disasters. *Psychiatric Annals, 15,* 153-155, 159-160.

Lipkin, J. O., Blank, A. S., & Scurfield, R. M. (1985). Forensic assessment of post-traumatic stress disorder in Viet Nam veterans. In S. M. Sonnenberg, A. S. Blank, & J. A. Talbott (Eds.), *The Trauma of War: Stress and Recovery in Viet Nam Veterans* (pp. 417-438). Washington, DC: American Psychiatric Press.

Lister, E. D. (1982, July). Forced silence: A neglected dimension of trauma. *American Journal of Psychiatry, 139,* 872-876.

Loftus, E., & Monahan, J. (1980, March). Trial by data: Psychological research as legal evidence. *American Psychologist, 35,* 270-283.

Martzke, J. S., Andersen, B. L., & Cacioppo, J. T. (1987). Cognitive assessment of anxiety disorders. In L. Michelson & L. M. Ascher (Eds.), *Anxiety and Stress Disorders: Cognitive-Behavioral Assessment and Treatment* (pp. 62-88). New York: Guilford.

McFarlane, A. C. (1986, January). Posttraumatic morbidity of a disaster: A study of cases presenting for psychiatric treatment. *Journal of Nervous and Mental Disease, 174,* 4-13.

McKenna, G. J., & Arthur, R. J. (1983). Survival under adverse conditions. *Directions in Psychiatry, 3* (Lesson 36), 1-7.

Modlin, H. C. (1967, February). The postaccident anxiety syndrome: Psychosocial aspects. *American Journal of Psychiatry, 123,* 1008-1012.

Modlin, H. C. (1983, December). Traumatic neurosis and other injuries. *Psychiatric Clinics of North America, 6,* 661-682.

Modlin, H. C. (1985). Is there an assault syndrome? *Bulletin of the American Academy of Psychiatry and the Law, 13,* 139-145.

Mueser, K. T., & Butler, R. W. (1987, March). Auditory hallucinations in combat-related chronic posttraumatic stress disorder. *American Journal of Psychiatry, 144,* 299-302.

Muse, M. (1986, June). Stress-related posttraumatic chronic pain syndrome: Behavioral treatment approach. *Pain, 25,* 389-394.

Nadelson, C. C., Notman, M. T., Zackson, H., & Gornick, J. (1982, October). A follow-up study of rape victims. *American Journal of Psychiatry, 139,* 1266-1270.

Newman, C. J. (1976, March). Children of disaster: Clinical observations at Buffalo Creek. *American Journal of Psychiatry, 133,* 306-312.

Notman, M. T., & Nadelson, C. C. (1976, April). The rape victim: Psychodynamic considerations. *American Journal of Psychiatry, 133,* 408-413.

Pina, G., III. (1985). Diagnosis and treatment of posttraumatic stress disorder in Hispanic Viet Nam veterans. In S. M. Sonnenberg, A. S. Blank, & J. A. Talbott (Eds.), *The Trauma of War: Stress and Recovery in Viet Nam Veterans* (pp. 389-402). Washington, DC: American Psychiatric Press.

Rangell, L. (1976, March). Discussion of the Buffalo Creek disaster: The course of psychic trauma. *American Journal of Psychiatry, 133,* 313-316.

Ravenscroft, K. (1982, August). The burn unit. *Psychiatric Clinics of North America, 5,* 419-432.

Reid, W. H. (1985, August). The antisocial personality: A review. *Hospital and Community Psychiatry, 36,* 831-837.

Rome, H. P. (1984, July). Reflections on traumatology. *Psychiatric Annals, 11,* 493.

Rose, D. S. (1986, July). "Worse than death": Psychodynamics of rape victims and the need for psychotherapy. *American Journal of Psychiatry, 143,* 817-824.

Rothschild, A. J. (1984). Acute grief: Disaster victims. In S. E. Hyman (Ed.), *Manual of Psychiatric Emergencies* (pp. 107-112). Boston: Little, Brown & Co.

Santiago, J. M., McCall-Perez, F., Gorcey, M., & Beigel, A. (1985, November). Long-term psychological effects of rape in 35 rape victims. *American Journal of Psychiatry, 142,* 1338-1340.

Schnaper, N., & Cowley, R. A. (1976, August). Overview: Psychiatric sequelae to multiple trauma. *American Journal of Psychiatry, 133,* 883-890.

Schottenfeld, R. S., & Cullen, M. R. (1985, February). Occupation-induced posttraumatic stress disorders. *American Journal of Psychiatry, 142,* 198-202.

Scrignar, C. B. (1987, July). Post-traumatic stress disorder. *The Psychiatric Times, 4*(7), 1, 8-11.

Scurfield, R. M., & Blank, A. S. (1985). A guide to obtaining a military history from Viet Nam veterans. In S. M. Sonnenberg, A. S. Blank, & J. A. Talbott (Eds.), *The Trauma of War: Stress and Recovery in Viet Nam Veterans* (pp. 263-292). Washington, DC: American Psychiatric Press.

Shatan, C. F. (1982, November). The tattered ego of survivors. *Psychiatric Annals, 12,* 1031-1038.

Shealy, C. N. (1984, Fall-Winter). Total life stress and symptomatology. *Journal of Holistic Medicine, 6,* 112-129.

Shore, J. H., Tatum, E. L., & Vollmer, W. M. (1986, May). Psychiatric reactions to disaster: The Mount St. Helens experience. *American Journal of Psychiatry, 143,* 590-595.

Sierles, F. S., Chen, J-J, McFarland, R. E., & Taylor, M. A. (1983, September). Posttraumatic stress disorder and concurrent psychiatric illness: A preliminary report. *American Journal of Psychiatry, 140,* 1177-1179.

Silver, S. M. (1985). Post-traumatic stress disorders in veterans. In P. A. Keller & L. G. Ritt (Eds.), *Innovations in Clinical Practice: A Source Book* (Vol. 4, pp. 23-34). Sarasota, FL: Professional Resource Exchange.

Singer, M. T. (1981, March). Viet Nam prisoners of war, stress, and personality resiliency. *American Journal of Psychiatry, 138,* 345-346.

Smith, J. R. (1982, November). Personal responsibility in traumatic stress reactions. *Psychiatric Annals, 12,* 1021-1025, 1029-1030.

Solomon, Z., & Benbenishty, R. (1986, May). The role of proximity, immediacy, and expectancy in frontline treatment of combat stress reaction among Israelis in the Lebanon War. *American Journal of Psychiatry, 143,* 613-617.

Solomon, Z., Garb, R., Bleich, A., & Grupper, D. (1987a, January). Reactivation of combat-related posttraumatic stress disorder. *American Journal of Psychiatry, 144,* 51-55.

Solomon, Z., Weisenberg, M., Schwarzwald, J., & Mikulincer, M. (1987b, April). Posttraumatic stress disorder among frontline soldiers with combat stress reaction: The 1982 Israeli experience. *American Journal of Psychiatry, 144,* 448-454.

Sonnenberg, S. M., Blank, A. S., & Talbott, J. A. (Eds.). (1985). *The Trauma of War: Stress and Recovery in Viet Nam Veterans.* Washington, DC: American Psychiatric Press.

Sparr, L. F., & Atkinson, R. M. (1986, May). Post-traumatic stress disorder as an insanity defense: Medicolegal quicksand. *American Journal of Psychiatry, 143,* 608-612.

Sparr, L., & Pankratz, L. D. (1983, August). Factitious posttraumatic stress disorder. *American Journal of Psychiatry, 140,* 1016-1019.

Stern, G. M. (1976, March). From chaos to responsibility. *American Journal of Psychiatry, 133,* 300-301.

Stone, M. H. (1986). Borderline personality disorder. In A. M. Cooper, A. J. Frances, & M. H. Sacks (Eds.), *Psychiatry* (Vol. 1): *The Personality Disorders and Neuroses* (pp. 203-217). New York: Basic Books.

Taylor, S. E. (1983, November). Adjustment to threatening events: A theory of cognitive adaptation. *American Psychologist, 38,* 1161-1173.

Tennant, C. C., Goulston, K. J., & Dent, O. F. (1986, May). The psychological effects of being a prisoner of war:

Forty years after release. *American Journal of Psychiatry, 143,* 618-621.

Thompson, G. N. (1965, May). Post-traumatic psycho-neurosis--A statistical survey. *American Journal of Psychiatry, 121,* 1043-1048.

Titchener, J. L., & Kapp, F. T. (1976, March). Family and character change at Buffalo Creek. *American Journal of Psychiatry, 133,* 295-299.

Ursano, R. J. (1981, March). The Viet Nam era prisoner of war: Precaptivity personality and the development of psychiatric illness. *American Journal of Psychiatry, 138,* 315-318.

Ursano, R. J., Boydstun, J. A., & Wheatley, R. D. (1981, March). Psychiatric illness in U. S. Air Force Viet Nam prisoners of war: A five-year follow-up. *American Journal of Psychiatry, 138,* 310-314.

van der Kolk, B. A. (1987, July). Trauma and psychiatric illness. *The Psychiatric Times, 4,* 5-6.

Van Dyke, C., Zilberg, N. J., & McKinnon, J. A. (1985, September). Posttraumatic stress disorder: A thirty-year delay in a World War II veteran. *American Journal of Psychiatry, 142,* 1070-1073.

Walker, J. I., & Cavenar, J. O. (1982, March). Vietnam veterans: Their problems continue. *Journal of Nervous and Mental Disease, 170,* 174-180.

Weissman, H. N. (1984, July). Psychological assessment and psycho-legal formulations in psychiatric traumatology. *Psychiatric Annals, 11,* 517-521, 525, 527-529.

West, L. J., & Coburn, K. (1984). Posttraumatic anxiety. In R. O. Pasnau (Ed.), *Diagnosis and Treatment of Anxiety Disorders* (pp. 81-113). Washington, DC: American Psychiatric Press.

Wilkinson, C. B. (1983, September). Aftermath of a disaster: The collapse of the Hyatt Regency Hotel skywalks. *American Journal of Psychiatry, 140,* 1134-1139.

Wilkinson, C. B. (1985, March). Introduction: The psychological consequences of disasters. *Psychiatric Annals, 15,* 135, 138-139.

Wilkinson, C. B., & Vera, E. (1985, March). The management and treatment of disaster victims. *Psychiatric Annals, 15,* 174-177, 180-181, 184.

Wilmer, H. A. (1982, November). Post-traumatic stress disorder. *Psychiatric Annals, 12,* 995, 998-1003.

Ziskin, J. (1981a). Cross-examination in personal injury cases. In *Coping with Psychiatric and Psychological*

Testimony (Vol. 2, 3rd ed., pp. 128-137). Venice, CA: Law and Psychology Press.

Ziskin, J. (1981b). Deficiencies in assessment of malingering or credibility. In *Coping with Psychiatric and Psychological Testimony* (Vol. 1, 3rd ed., pp. 429-441). Venice, CA: Law and Psychology Press.

Ziskin, J. (1981c). Appendix B. A personal injury case. In *Coping with Psychiatric and Psychological Testimony* (Vol. 2, 3rd ed., pp. 172-202). Venice, CA: Law and Psychology Press.

3.

Post-Traumatic Stress Disorder: Differential Diagnosis

Herbert C. Modlin

Post-traumatic stress disorder (PTSD) in pure form is one of the most specific diagnostic categories in current psychiatric nomenclature, and differential diagnosis poses few problems. The cardinal symptoms of anxiety, repetitive nightmares, flashbacks, startle reaction, and phobic avoidance of circumstances related to the traumatic event, when they occur together, are not diagnostically characteristic of any other mental disorder (Modlin, 1986). Unfortunately, many patients do not present "pure" clinical syndromes to fit the neat labels in the revised third edition of the *Diagnostic and Statistical Manual of Mental Disorders* (*DSM-III-R*; American Psychiatric Association, 1987). Problems in differential diagnosis do arise because (a) PTSD patients commonly present additional symptoms such as restlessness, fatigue, insomnia, difficulty in concentration and memory, loss of sexual capacity, and social withdrawal, all of which familiarly accompany other illnesses; (b) the full PTSD syndrome may not develop in every patient; and (c) various other disorders, such as depression, substance abuse, antisocial behavior, cerebral concussion, or brief psychotic episodes, may be concomitant with PTSD and smudge the diagnostic canvas.

This chapter will detail the differentiation of PTSD from generalized anxiety disorder, panic disorder, major depressive episode, and post-concussion syndrome. Accurate diagnosis, to the extent that present knowledge allows, is important in that treatment, disability, and prognosis differ for the various disorders.

GENERALIZED ANXIETY DISORDER

The four characteristic features of generalized anxiety disorder (GAD) are anxious expectation, muscle tension, vigilant scanning, and autonomic nervous system activity (Barlow, 1985). Autonomic nervous system overactivity (tight chest, heart palpitations, sweating, nausea, diarrhea, urinary frequency) is rare in PTSD, but the other three features are frequent components.

Apprehensive expectation in GAD is manifestly unrealistic anxiety and worry about ordinary life circumstances: unfounded fear of job loss, irrational concern over finances, or apprehension about physical illness in the face of good health. The common denominator in such exaggerated concerns is double barreled, a loss of self-reliance and of reasonable trust in one's environment leading to a sense of helplessness.

Muscle tension is demonstrated by trembling, restlessness, easy fatigability, and sudden starts, usually when drifting off to sleep. Hypervigilance is mostly self-explanatory, but besides being recognizable in wary scanning of the environment (and one's self) for possible dangers, it is characterized by a startle reaction to unexpected noises, difficulty with concentration and memory, insomnia, and a general feeling of being keyed up or on edge.

The characteristic symptoms of the disorder may appear in any clinical syndrome in which anxiety is a prominent component. A diagnosis of true GAD rests in part on exclusion. If there are no panic attacks, no anxious obsessive-compulsive ruminations, no significant agitated depression, no frightening thoughts of suicide, none of the basic symptoms of PTSD, then the diagnosis of generalized anxiety disorder can be established. There may be troublesome dreams but they are not related to a specific, real, potentially life-threatening event as in PTSD. The patient may report scary dreams of falling, of swimming in a boundless ocean, or of seeing a vague, threatening figure.

The *DSM-III-R* suggests that the symptoms should remain for at least 6 months. This stipulation is in effect to insure separation of GAD from episodes of normal anxiety or situational adjustment disorder related to a real problem that may seem to be unmanageable for a period. The onset of GAD may coincide with some life event that is eventually settled or resolved, while the apprehension it aroused inappropriately lingers. The condition remains chronic; it is not episodic, although the intensity of symptoms may fluctuate.

It should be noted, in passing, that GAD may be secondary to some physical disorder, such as hyperthyroidism, hypoglycemia, or substance abuse reactions (McNeil, 1987).

Consider the following case example:

A.B., a 32-year-old housewife and the mother of 5- and 7-year-old girls, was involved in a minor intersection "fender bender." She was emotionally shaken by the experience, particularly when she discovered that she had passed a stop sign (unseen by her) and was responsible for the accident. Never a confident driver, she became quite apprehensive while driving, especially if accompanied by her daughters. Her concern spread: She worried about the girls walking home from school - "something could happen"; she worried that the accident would cause the car insurance to be canceled. She became chronically tense, had difficulty sleeping, and neglected housework because of fatigue. At the market, she forgot what she was to purchase. Her husband joshed her at first for her ridiculous fears, then grew irritated, intensifying her insecurity.

When seen for clinical evaluation 8 months post-accident, she described her many symptoms, reiterating, "I know it's silly, but . . . ." Questioning revealed that she had experienced a similar episode during her first year at college, which resulted in her leaving school and seeking therapy.

PANIC DISORDER

Panic disorder is a discrete, episodic experience of overwhelming anxiety with relatively normal periods between attacks. The onset is usually sudden and attacks occur, with no apparent precipitating stimulus, at any time of the day or night, such as when driving, at the work desk, or in the kitchen. Characteristically, the episodes take place one or more times a week and subside within hours or, at most, a day. The "normal" interepisode period of some patients is beset by chronic uneasiness, mild agoraphobia, and apprehension about the next acute attack (Nemiah, 1984).

The primary symptoms of panic attacks are as follows:

1. Onset of acute, painful anxiety even to the point of terror and fear of dying.
2. Striking "cardiac" symptoms of chest pain, constricted breathing, and heart palpitations. The pain may mimic a real anginal attack by radiating into the left arm.
3. Additional somatic symptoms such as flushing, sweating, trembling, lump in the throat, and tingling in the hands and feet.
4. Disturbances of consciousness with dizziness, swimming sensations, faintness, and mental confusion.
5. Feelings of unreality or of going "crazy."

Again, in "pure" form the differential diagnosis between panic attacks and PTSD is usually clear. However, both syndromes can occur together or, more commonly, once PTSD develops, panic attacks may be a complicating sequel and the clinical picture, including thoughts about treatment, becomes muddled.

As noted in the preceding section, GAD shares some symptoms with panic attack, but the former is chronic, relatively unremitting, and of low intensity, whereas the latter is episodic, with relief periods, and is of high intensity. The following case is illustrative.

C.D., a 30-year-old married man with one child, was an installer of satellite TV dishes weighing several hundred pounds each. On one occasion, his co-worker let go of a dish, which came down on C.D. and threatened to crush him. By a superhuman effort, he shoved the dish to one side, but his hand was mashed, requiring amputation of the thumb. While recuperating from surgery, he repetitively suffered nightmares reproducing the falling dish. As it was about to strike him, he would waken with a yell, rousing his wife. He become tense, anxious, and irritable; developed a startle reaction to sharp noises; slept fitfully and paced restlessly; and lost interest in marital sex.

Eventually C.D. returned to his job, but was fired when he refused to go near a dish. His wife found employment, which furthered his discouragement and low self-esteem. His depression was deepened by mourning over his lost thumb. Through efforts of his attorney, he sought help at the State Vocational Rehabilitation Service where a counselor discovered his talent for drawing and placed him with a machine manufacturing company in an office job as blueprint assistant to two engineers. He liked the job; his tension eased and the nightmares subsided. However, he had to walk through the shop frequently between noisy, banging, moving machines. He experienced tension, shakiness, perspiration, and faint feelings. While driving home one evening, he developed overwhelming anxiety, hyperventilation, heart palpitations, severe constricting chest pain, mental clouding, and weakness. He stopped until his thoughts and vision cleared, then went to a hospital emergency room with his "heart attack." Findings of the examination were entirely normal, as were his family physician's the next day.

An exact recurrence of symptoms three nights later sent him to the hospital again. Following four such attacks in 3 weeks, his physician referred him for psychiatric evaluation. After several sessions with explanation, support, reassurance, and excellent response to antianxiety medication, he was able to return to work. A short while later, he was afforded the opportunity to move to an architectural firm quite free of machinery. He had no more attacks. However, he is a quieter man than before, does not care to socialize, still flares up over trivial matters, and only occasionally can experience sexual arousal.

MAJOR DEPRESSIVE EPISODE

The current nosological labels for affective disorders are bipolar disorder, major depression, and dysthymic disorder (neurotic depression). Affect is a term used to denote a strong, abnormal feeling of depression or elation that pervades the whole psychic life and influences thought and behavior. Approximate synonyms are feeling, emotion, and mood, but those terms also indicate such experiences as anger, rage, love, and loneliness.

Bipolar refers to an illness in which the moods of elation and euphoria alternate with those of depression and despondency, often with relatively normal periods between episodes. The two states are opposite poles of emotions run rampant. There is frequently a family history of the illness, and it is based, in part, on an abnormality of brain chemistry.

An episode of major depression may occur only once in the life of a patient, or it may be recurrent, but manic episodes never occur. The symptoms required to establish the diagnosis are depressed mood, lessened interest and pleasure in activities, weight loss or gain, insomnia or hypersomnia, motor agitation or retardation, fatigue, feelings of guilt or worthlessness, impaired concentration or attention, and thoughts of death or suicide. Psychotic episodes with delusions and hallucinations are possible but are infrequent (McNeil, 1987).

Depressed patients do not complain of frightening nightmares or daytime flashbacks related to a specific real-life event, nor do they mention startle reaction or other cardinal symptoms of anxiety disorders such as PTSD. The "depression" in PTSD patients is usually an understandable discouragement related to realistic problems such as work disability, handicapping physical illness, lessened income, marital friction, or loss of self-esteem.

Dysthymic disorder is described in the *DSM-III-R* as having symptoms nearly identical to those of major depression, and a clinical choice between the two nosological labels may be problematic. Dysthymic disorder is chronic and unremitting in contrast to a major depressive episode, lasting for years. Some authorities have considered it a personality disorder (Kocsis & Frances, 1987). Some individuals may evidence symptoms of more than one diagnosis. The following case illustrates such a dual diagnosis.

E.F., 18, was driving back to college with her long-time best friend as a passenger. She swerved to avoid a car and was hit head-on by a semi-trailer truck. She landed in the road feeling panicky and confused. She was transported by ambulance to a hospital, where examination disclosed a fractured femur, low back pain, and multiple cuts and bruises. The 3-weeks' hospital stay was largely a blur because of the medications. She learned that her friend had died in the wreck. At home she had frightening dreams reproducing the accident, slept fitfully, and became tense, fatigued, irritable, and withdrawn. Concentration was impaired and she could not read with comprehension. She gained 35 pounds as a result of her frequent nibbling.

E.F. remained depressed and in mourning for her friend. She visited the grave frequently and cried. She refused to drive, and when she was a passenger, she was a vociferous backseat driver. Her mother described with feeling her daughter's irritability and temper flare-ups, her "impossible" attitude in a car, and her considerable depression.

When evaluated 2 years post-accident at the request of her attorney, E.F. reported cessation of the nightmares, but continuing tension, irritability, and apprehension in a car. She had just experienced a bad "anniversary" reaction to the death of her friend 2 years earlier with thoughts of self-blame. She was discouraged over the loss of her planned college career. She had returned to school, but could not study, failed tests, and quit. She obtained a job but was fired for slowness and errors. Her present job was going better.

In this case, two concurrent diagnoses seemed indicated: PTSD and depression. A differential between major depression and bereavement is difficult to determine since the diagnostic picture is complicated by the PTSD symptoms. The "anniversary" reaction argues for bereavement (McNeil, 1987).

POST-CONCUSSION SYNDROME

A blow to the head may produce variable consequences, from minor to serious to lethal. Since the brain is encased in bone, a sharp head blow can make the brain shake briefly, like a bowl of jelly, and bounce against the skull. A frequent result is cerebral concussion with no skull fracture (closed head injury) but a brief period of unconsciousness, usually only of some minutes' duration, and subsequent amnesia. There is no brain laceration or blood clot, but tiny microscopic hemorrhages and damage to individual nerve cells can occur. Usually these changes are reversible and concussion is a recoverable illness.

Nine symptoms of the post-concussion syndrome have been described: headache, dizzy spells, irritability, nervousness, impaired concentration, confusion, optic symptoms, fatigue, and alcohol intolerance (Long & Webb, 1983). Difficulties with concentration and attention, nervousness, irritability, and fatigue are familiar components of PTSD; and headaches and periods of confusion occur occasionally. The differential diagnosis can pose questions, particularly if both conditions develop concurrently from the same accident. Individuals with post-concussion syndrome may, therefore, also evidence the complete PTSD symptom complex, as the following case illustrates.

G.H., 25, a construction worker, was hit on the head by a swinging crane boom and knocked down. He stood up feeling groggy, only to be hit again by the boom. He was briefly unconscious and was taken to a hospital emergency room, where findings from physical examination and x-rays were negative. He was told that he had a concussion and should see his family doctor.

He returned to work in a few days but was so confused, nervous, and apprehensive that he quit and went home. He became quite nervous, irritable, forgetful, and withdrawn. He had persistent severe headaches and difficulty focusing his eyes. He experienced disturbing feelings of derealization in which he felt detached from reality and had nightmares of "things" coming at him out of the dark. He was depressed and tearful, apprehensive about leaving home, and very dependent on his wife.

Neurological test findings, including an electroencephalogram (EEG) and head computerized axial tomography (CAT) scan, were negative. The psychiatrist noted the typical PTSD symptoms but was puzzled by the severe concentration impairment, the derealization phenomena, and G.H.'s collapse into helplessness. The internist at the headache clinic diagnosed post-concussion headache but raised the question of psychogenic factors.

A neurological test battery 3 months post-accident revealed definite organic deficits, including a reduced ability to concentrate, to remember, and to react normally to environmental stimuli. The concussed brain does not process incoming information well (Trimble, 1981). G.H. was treated with analgesics, antianxiety medication, and supportive psychotherapy. A repeat test battery 7 months post-accident revealed marked improvement in brain function. Most of the PTSD symptoms had resolved and he was able to obtain employment at a gas station. He refused to return to construction work.

G.H. sustained a cerebral concussion of some severity as well as a PTSD and a secondary depression. With remission of the organic impairment, he regained most of his former competence. With the help of psychotherapy, he relinquished his comfortable dependence and ventured into the world again.

Long and Webb (1983) report a study of 129 patients who suffered minor head injuries: 87% manifested impairment on the neuropsychological tests while only 29% had an abnormal EEG and 26% a positive CAT scan. Given the fact of a normal neurological examination, many clinicians will conclude that the patient's symptoms are psychogenic. Some are, including a full-blown PTSD, but the subtle impact of a post-concussion syndrome should be considered.

In addition to professional experience and expert clinical acumen, some useful adjuncts to the diagnostic interview can be considered. Some clinicians use rating scales for depression, anxiety, and other disorders, and find them useful as a checklist. Such scales should be supplemental to a good clinical evaluation as they do not reflect the all important factor of personal patient-clinician interchange or the operation of the clinical inference process. Since most PTSD patients are also legal clients (personal injury suits, workers' compensation claims), the attorney can be a useful source of ancillary data by supplying school, military, work, or medical records, as the case dictates. A spouse or other close person should be interviewed to confirm the patient's account and to check on possible exaggerations or omissions in his or her story. Problems of overreaction, secondary gain, and even malingering need to be kept in mind.

Herbert C. Modlin, MD, received an honorable DSc degree from the University of Nebraska and did post-graduate work in psychiatry and neurology in Philadelphia, Boston, and Montreal (1940-1943). He was Chief of Neuropsychiatric Services at the Topeka VA Hospital in 1946-1949 and has been a staff member at the Menninger Clinic since 1949. He was a candidate at the Topeka Psychoanalytic Institute from 1947-1954. Dr. Modlin is board certified in psychiatry, neurology, and forensic psychiatry, and is a past President of the American Board of Forensic Psychiatry. He currently is a Professor of Forensic Psychiatry at the Menninger School of Psychiatry, and a visiting lecturer at the University of Kansas Medical School and Law School. His special interests include personal injury, stress response syndromes, and disaster syndromes, and he has numerous publications in these areas. Dr. Modlin can be reached at The Menninger Clinic, Box 829, Topeka, KS 66601-0829.

REFERENCES

American Psychiatric Association. (1987). *Diagnostic and Statistical Manual of Mental Disorders* (3rd ed. rev.). Washington, DC: Author.

Barlow, D. (1985). The dimensions of anxiety disorders. In H. Tuma & J. Maser (Eds.), *Anxiety and the Anxiety Disorders* (p. 492). Hillsdale, NJ: Lawrence Erlbaum Associates.

Kocsis, J., & Frances, A. (1987). A critical discussion of *DSM-III* dysthymic disorder. *American Journal of Psychiatry, 144*, 1534-1542.

Long, C., & Webb, W. (1983). Psychological sequelae of head trauma. *Psychiatric Medicine, 1*, 33-37.

McNeil, G. (1987). Anxiety. In S. Soreff & G. McNeil (Eds.), *Handbook of Differential Diagnosis* (pp. 20-32). Littleton, MA: PSG Publishing Co.

Modlin, H. (1986). Post-traumatic stress disorder. *Postgraduate Medicine, 79*, 26-48.

Nemiah, J. (1984). Neurotic disorders. In H. Kaplan & B. Sadock (Eds.), *Comprehensive Textbook of Psychiatry* (pp. 889-891). Baltimore: Williams & Wilkins.

Trimble, M. (1981). *Posttraumatic Neurosis*. New York: John Wiley & Sons.

4.

Social Factors Associated with Post-Traumatic Stress Disorder in Vietnam Veterans

Herbert J. Cross

One benefit of the costly Vietnam conflict was the impetus for social science to understand the effects of great stress on a large number of people. The concept of post-traumatic stress disorder (PTSD) is more closely linked to the Vietnam era than to other associated phenomena such as rape, assault, and natural or human-made disasters.

Much of the relevant literature is cited in Figley's (1985) recent work. Figley is a Vietnam veteran and one of the most active professionals writing about PTSD. The inclusion of PTSD as a specific diagnostic entity in the American Psychiatric Association's (1980) *Diagnostic and Statistical Manual of Mental Disorders* (*DSM-III*) was partly based on the disorder presented by many veterans. Prior to *DSM-III*, the most similar entity in the *DSM-II* (American Psychiatric Association, 1968) was classified under "adjustment reactions of adult life," where combat stress was mentioned under "Adult Adjustment Reaction: fear associated with military combat and manifested by trembling, running, and hiding" (*DSM-II*, American Psychiatric Association, 1968, cited in Figley, 1978). The original *Diagnostic and Statistical Manual of Mental Disorders* (*DSM-I*, American Psychiatric Association, 1952) defined a class of gross stress reactions as situations in which the individual had been exposed to severe physical demands or extreme emotional stress, including combat situations (Figley, 1978, p. xvii).

During the Korean War, the Department of the Navy used the term "combat fatigue"; in World War II, the term was "battle fatigue," and in World War I, "shell shock." The shell-shock syndrome of World War I was thought to have been based on the shock to the nervous system of the sound of exploding shells, especially relevant in a war of established defenses and artillery barrages. In the late 1800s, compensation laws had given rise to lawsuits against railroads for "railway spine," the diagnosis of which was promulgated by a British professor of surgery, John Erichsen (1882), who believed that the shock of railway jolts contributed to concussion of the spine and to nervous symptoms.

Because these early conceptualizations were related to compensation, the term "compensation neurosis" and the concepts of "secondary gain" and malingering were associated with the new diagnosis. Secondary gain is an orthodox psychoanalytic concept that suggests that patients unconsciously benefit from symptoms and, therefore, perpetuate them. Malingering, of course, is despised as dishonest and illegal. Another aspect of psychoanalysis that has affected conceptualization of PTSD is the notion of predisposition. Psychoanalysis has generally promoted the view that all neurotic symptoms have roots in an individual's developmental history. Therefore, any "neurotic" reaction to an environmental stressor would inevitably involve a strong predisposition.

These psychoanalytic influences, plus a long association with suspected malingering and cowardice, help to stigmatize any field soldier who cannot fight because of combat fatigue. The affected battle casualty, then, is partly to blame for the disorder. Such a casualty might be described in the troops' vernacular of Vietnam as a "non-hacker" (i.e., one who could not "hack" the rigors of combat). Needless to say, such a stigma involves considerable personal discomfort.

Another aspect of PTSD is that it may not be manifested until months, or even years, after the precipitating stress. A disorder that shows an onset several years after the war still implies some deficit in the person or some special vulnerability that stigmatizes him or her as less effective than or simply not as tough as other veterans. Many veterans are reluctant to make a claim for such a disorder because they must admit to mental symptoms of distress. Put another way, they must declare that they are mentally impaired and are in need of assistance. Since claims for disability are not readily accepted, an involved and painful effort may be too strenuous for many who thus choose not to seek help even though they need it.

Therefore, PTSD is a problematic disorder for those who suffer from it over and above its symptoms, because the consequences are great. Further, since there is overlap with other categories and criteria are complex, the diagnosis is often unclear and problematic.

Because of the special nature of the Vietnam conflict and the turbulence of the 1960s in the United States, there are many factors associated with veteran status that contribute to PTSD or some aspect of dealing with it. Some of these factors will be discussed after a closer look at the nature of the disorder.

DESCRIPTION OF
POST-TRAUMATIC STRESS DISORDER

The *DSM-III* description served the function of supplying the syndrome with an official and relatively usable description. The disorder is not defined solely by symptoms, however, because the symptoms must follow an "... event that is outside the range of usual human experience" (American Psychiatric Association, 1980, p. 247). The inclusion of an environmental event in the diagnostic criteria seems limiting to some (Trimble, 1985) and clearly requires a difficult judgment. The symptoms involve three major aspects: a re-experience of the traumatic event, reduced responsiveness or numbing to the current environment, and several cognitive or autonomic symptoms that overlap with anxiety and depression. The characteristic that seems most unique to PTSD and that may fuel many other symptoms is the re-experiencing - which can be manifested in nightmarish dreams, intrusive memories, or obsessions about the trauma or some aspect of it. The PTSD patient, then, is not consciously free of the original trauma until this re-experiencing ceases and, by its very nature, re-experiencing does not seem to be under his or her control. Horowitz (1986) has discussed this aspect of PTSD in theoretical terms. He proposes that the initiating trauma is so foreign to the victim's assumptions about the world and his or her own identity that it cannot easily be integrated into his or her beliefs about reality. Many disaster and rape victims have stated their disbelief of the events as they were happening and later. Vietnam veterans also frequently state their amazement and disbelief at their experiences. In order to recover, the victim must somehow reintegrate his or her shattered assumptions of the world into a workable set of beliefs that allow some adaptive uses of mental faculties and relief from focus on the trauma.

This formulation is based on an information-processing model that should seem plausible to any cognitive psychologist (i.e., information input is ordinarily matched with old information and stored in the appropriate category for future reference or use). Information that is thoroughly deviant from the assumptions already held cannot be categorized easily. A painful process of re-examining assumptions about self-world, identity, and the nature of the world frequently produces emotions and thoughts that are maladaptive or debilitating. Vietnam veterans who have experienced trauma frequently cannot forget a particular scene (e.g., the sight of a man's face as part of his body is destroyed). The graphic replay of horror may continue until the reintegration can be made. If the person can avoid the traumatic situation or completely change his or her environment, as was possible for "mede-vacked" wounded (evacuated for medical reasons) in Vietnam, the ruminative re-experience may be suppressed so that the victim is unaware of it. This quick suppression of ruminative re-experiencing seems to be a likely antecedent to delayed stress symptoms that may become evident after 6 months. Symptoms that emerge months or years after the trauma are more difficult to treat and can be intensely upsetting for the victim.

The victim's serious discomfort is partly related to loss of control over his or her own mental processes. Recurrent images of horror, called "unbidden images" by Horowitz (1986), are frightening to most people because they can be likened to hallucinations and serious mental disorder. In other words, people who are depressed and anxious, and are disrupted by unbidden re-experiencing of their most negative memories, often think they are hopelessly "crazy" or are clearly on the way to debilitating mental illness. Therefore, PTSD is often a serious and incapacitating disorder. The *DSM-III* notes that severity seems greater when the trauma is of "human design" (e.g., war, torture, or rape). Perhaps the "human design" aspect of great trauma allows the victim to direct his or her rage at a perpetrator who is obviously blameworthy. It is more difficult to be enraged at the capriciousness of earthquakes, floods, and the like than at enemies; however, if enemies cannot be reached or punished, it seems even more difficult to accept the damage.

The numbing or constriction of affect is conceived by Horowitz (1986) and Shatan (1978) as related to the overwhelming arousal associated with the trauma and defending against the same. Many disaster victims and Vietnam veterans speak of being unable to feel or of having isolated themselves from their emotions. Horowitz also treats numbing as a phase of the disorder that must be worked through if the affected individual is to make progress toward a cure. Showing and feeling emotion are always difficult for a sufferer of any serious negative feeling. It is common knowledge that dwelling on past difficulties is maladaptive. However, the "numbing" of PTSD is so automatic and consistent that it seems unlikely to be a conscious mechanism of protection. It seems to be beyond the control of the sufferer and related to defensively protecting oneself from the devastating event. Lazarus and Golden (1981) believe that denial is a necessary and useful adaptation to stress. Taylor (1983) cites several authors who have concluded that people generally are more optimistic about themselves than is warranted by the data. It does seem likely that we ignore our faults and errors while emphasizing our strengths and successes. So, it seems that idealistic illusions are a component of everyday thinking. Of course, after one has been exposed to massive destruction, prolonged danger, or many deaths, illusory optimism seems impossible. Many Vietnam veterans speak of having lost their innocence or youthful optimism.

It seems likely that the numbing so frequently seen in response to great trauma is related to defending oneself psychologically against overwhelming information. The knowledge that others wish to humiliate you and torture you in the most horrible manner conceivable, or to kill you without the slightest hesitation, is exceptionally discomfiting information. Maintaining one's self-esteem in the face of such information is difficult. Once the fragility of life and the extent of cruelty are clearly experienced by an idealistic young person, numbing may be the only possible response.

The *DSM-III* revision (*DSM-III-R*, American Psychiatric Association, 1987) is more inclusive than its predecessor, but the major symptom patterns are the same, except that the active category has been eliminated.

Other symptoms of PTSD, such as rage, resentment, autonomic arousal, depression, and concentration difficulties, are less unique than re-experiencing intensive images or numbing, but they can be extremely debilitating and fearsome to the victim.

PROBLEMS WITH THE POST-TRAUMATIC STRESS DISORDER CONCEPT

Psychoanalytic conceptions of the effects of great stress have been mentioned. Grinker and Spiegel (1945) wrote the major study of the World War II era, which perpetuated psychoanalytic thinking about psychological effects of combat. The most important idea fostered by this work was that victims of combat stress were uniquely predisposed to their disorder. Once the notion of predisposition is accepted, then there is less need to focus on the nature of the stress, as it is only one factor in the outcome of disability. In other words, predisposed people have already progressed partway to their disorder and are partly to blame for it.

The concept of predisposition is controversial for Vietnam veterans because a focus on predisposition toward disorder furthers the idea that Vietnam veterans are partly to blame for their troubles. Veterans, then, are further stigmatized by attributing one more negative characteristic to them. If they were predisposed, then the war and government are less blameworthy.

One implication, then, is that the government is not responsible for offering services or compensation to these veterans. This is exactly the situation that existed until 1980 when PTSD was officially recognized as a diagnostic entity. Veterans who presented themselves as needing treatment in the late 1960s or early 1970s were frequently misdiagnosed, and even mistreated, because of the lack of professional understanding.

When the research that bears on the predisposition issue is reviewed (Boulanger, 1985), there is no clear-cut answer. One group of investigators attributed a good deal of influence to predisposing factors, but they did not adequately account for amount of combat experience (Robins, 1981). Boulanger noted that family stability interacts with the likelihood of developing PTSD, but that the most important single factor is the amount and severity of combat.

So the stigma of predisposition has had negative effects on veterans. Clinicians probably work much more effectively with Vietnam veterans if they do not emphasize predisposing factors in their treatment. Obviously, a useful attitude with which to approach veterans with PTSD is that every human is vulnerable and anyone can develop symptoms if he or she has been exposed to the proper circumstances.

PREVALENCE OF POST-TRAUMATIC STRESS DISORDER IN VIETNAM, KOREAN, AND WORLD WAR II VETERANS

Partly because of the psychoanalytic influence (Grinker & Spiegel, 1945) and partly because of the nature of the war, there was little focus on the disabling effects on veterans after World War II. The war was strongly supported by society and victory reinforced a national image of invincibility and world leadership. The most comprehensive research done on service personnel, *The American Soldier* (Stouffer et al., 1949), focused on the efficiency of combat units, not on the experiences of combatants. We have discovered since World War II that many combatants suffered a syndrome essentially similar to Vietnam veterans' PTSD. World War II combat stress figures are estimated at about 10%, while Korean war figures are estimated to be 4% and comparable figures for Vietnam were estimated to be about 1% (Bourne, 1970). However, approximately one-third of Vietnam veterans are believed to show symptoms of PTSD (Williams, 1980). Whatever the inaccuracies in these figures are, it is clear that Vietnam had an astonishingly severe impact on the individuals who fought there even though the combat evacuations were slight. An exploration of some of the reasons is warranted, although the topic deserves more attention than is possible here.

THE VIETNAM TRAUMA

During the period of the Vietnam combat, American culture changed at a more rapid rate than ever before. Major attitudinal shifts with respect to hedonism, respect for tradition, and generational conflict were observed (Cross & Kleinhesselink, 1985). The war was a major focus for the youth of America. Everyone of draft age was affected. Recreational drug use, greater sexual freedom, and a youthful distrust of established institutions were related to attitudes about the war. Young men who were drafted or who volunteered under the pressure of the draft frequently were ambivalent about themselves because they believed that the draft was inequitable and that those with advantages were not drafted. In many ways, the stigma of being a Vietnam veteran began with the preinduction decision to face the "military obligation" rather than to feign illness or leave the country. As the war continued, there was more evidence that the American people were not supportive of the armed forces (Summers, 1982). The U.S. government's policy, never clear and unwavering, became obviously flawed as personnel and supply problems increased and public sentiment for withdrawal grew. The effect of these factors on the combatants was great. An already poorly directed war became worse. Leadership from field-grade officers was poor (Baritz, 1985), military discipline gave way to expediency, and the use of intoxicants was dangerously high. For example, a veteran who was a radio operator stated that he always kept a hash pipe in the radio shack because, "I knew that if I did my job, nobody cared, and besides that, I was already in the worst place they could send me."

In addition to the social factors and abortive military policy, a tropical jungle is the worst imaginable place to fight a guerrilla war, especially for those who grew up with clean sheets and plumbing. The climate, insects, snakes, rats, and tropical diseases were more than mere inconveniences. An infantry veteran related the following: "We were all interested when we found this ball of tiny snakes. There were hundreds. Then we got spooked when we realized that they were cobras and mama had to be close around."

The enemy was formidable, fighting on his own territory, mostly invisible or indistinguishable from the South Vietnamese, and able to sustain an incredible number of casualties without weakening. There was really little that favored the American forces except modern weapons and air power. The limited tours of duty (for the army, 12 months; the marines, 13 months) and the system of sending individuals as replacements undermined unit morale and the *esprit de corps* that had been noted in other wars, because people went as strangers to already operating units. Rarely were whole units sent to Vietnam after the buildup of 1966. Consequently, the DEROs (date of expected return from overseas) was uppermost in each individual's mind. The war was over for a soldier when the soldier's time was over. Efficiency was hampered because combat veterans did not wish to rely on "FNGs" (fucking new guys) who were not fully integrated until they had survived an initiation period. Near the end of a tour, less than 2 months remaining brought "short-timer" status where less was expected of someone who was almost ready to leave. In some units, short timers were not expected to do dangerous duty, and some line companies even sent short timers to rear echelons. These procedures contributed to an individual survival attitude that helped to undercut cooperation and unit morale. As the system fostered individuality, it supported prejudice against Asians and competition between Blacks and Whites, as well as distance between officers and enlisted personnel.

As the war continued, particularly after the Tet offensive of 1968, military efficiency declined and individual troops' resentment probably increased, as suggested by "fragging" (endangering or killing officers with fragmentation grenades), "sandbagging" (pretending to patrol but remaining in safer territory), increased use of intoxicants, and discipline problems. Cooperation with the South Vietnamese was frequently a problem and the ubiquitous dishonesty and corruption fostered callousness. Further, in the last 5 years of the war, most enlisted personnel were exposed to a mounting peace movement and antiwar sentiments in the United States, so that their preinduction experiences probably made them less prepared to fight and more reluctant to die for a cause that was questionably just and already lost.

Furthermore, the troops were not ignorant of weakening U.S. government support for the war. Much of this information was demoralizing because a major message was that the effort they expended and the danger they faced were for little yield.

Many veterans related the idea that Vietnam was surrealistic, that events moved too fast and made a great impact, but were devoid of meaning. It seems likely that this notion of meaninglessness was one of the great differences between Vietnam and previous wars. It simply did not make sense to say that one was fighting to save the world from communism, or for freedom for the South Vietnamese. The war was too confusing and the enemy was too ephemeral to focus upon as the cause of it all.

Meaningfulness, or commitment to a worthy cause, is thought to ameliorate the effects of great stress (Frankl, 1962). Veterans frequently report that the loss of comrades and other disturbing events were exacerbated because they had no real meaning.

Another particularly pathogenic factor in the Vietnam combat was the age of the combatants. In World War II, the average age of military personnel was about 26; in Vietnam, it was about 19.5. It has been noted that young people are easier to conscript, to train, and to induce to fight than are older people (LaBarre, 1954). It has also been noted that the young seem to suffer more from the experience (Jurich, 1983). Young people who are taken from their usual developmental tasks are hampered in acquiring the skills needed for adult life in a competitive society. The late teen years are characteristically a time for education and job training, as well as learning to relate to members of the opposite sex in a manner that allows effective mating and family life. Combat job skills do not transfer easily to practice and most young military men relate to foreign women in a manner that does not facilitate long-term mating and family life. Thus, there were a number of factors that seemed to increase the likelihood of PTSD in Vietnam veterans over and above those experienced in other wars.

THE POST-TRAUMATIC STRESS DISORDER-RESENTMENT CONTINUUM

Kormos (1978) defined acute combat reaction as a rejection of the role of combatant. His conceptualization is congruent with current knowledge about PTSD. Resentment toward commanding officers or toward the entire military system seems likely for any individual who has experienced PTSD associated with combat. Therefore, it seems fruitful to regard veterans' resentment of authority as related to the same conditions that are associated with PTSD. Horowitz (1974) noted that PTSD victims often alternate between intense feelings of sadness, grief, and rage at the people whom they blame for this distress. Vietnam veterans express anger most frequently at the U.S. government, their immediate field commanders, and the enemy.

Veterans' resentment toward the government seems partly fueled by their adjustment difficulties and frustrations. Since the government is in charge, it is a focus of anger. The development of anger and resentment might proceed as follows: A disgruntled, fearful, and uncertain soldier participates in or witnesses a traumatic scene that arouses him greatly. The government is involved because the government caused him to be at the scene. In Vietnam, errors by field commanders were frequent. When the stress traumas were clearly linked to command error, troop resentment was exceptionally high. One veteran expressed anger toward a new commanding officer (CO) who had just transferred in from an artillery unit. Because the officer wanted to give his old unit a chance to shell the enemy, he did not advance as was warranted, allowing a counterattack and much loss of American life. The veteran was so enraged that 16 years later he could not talk of the battle without screaming hatred for the CO. This veteran's symptoms were accompanied by feelings of anger and helplessness. Since the cause of the trauma was a government official, the veteran is angry at the government for causing the trauma, and for doing little to treat his disorder.

Distressed Vietnam veterans frequently express resentment at the government that ordered them to serve in Vietnam. Perhaps they more frequently express anger toward the Veterans Administration (VA) for failing to aid them with their disabilities or to provide treatment. One veteran noted that one has to be so well put together to jump all the VA hurdles that anyone with the least amount of irrationality could never do it. Certainly, veterans with low frustration tolerance, many of whom are alienated from all social institutions, have strong beliefs that the VA does not wish to help them. They will not pursue claims for disability for a number of reasons. Some, they state, are as follows: The screening procedure is designed to frustrate you so you will drop your claim. The appointments are arbitrarily set, with no regard for travel costs, employment, or convenience. Further, once a PTSD claim has been approved, the pension will likely be cut or disallowed if adjustment success is shown, such as achievement in education or employment. In other words, the pension is difficult to obtain and the procedure entails great personal discomfort. Frequently, veterans regard the procedure as demeaning and classify it as another discriminatory act of the same government that sent them to fight an unjust war from a strategically untenable position.

The Agent Orange controversy (Wilcox, 1983) is another issue that has incited a good deal of mistrust among veterans. Agent Orange was a herbicide that was used in Vietnam to defoliate enemy hiding places and to contaminate enemy food supplies. Dioxin, the major component, is a deadly poison. There are many stories of veterans showing symptoms of poisoning who were treated poorly by the VA. Dangerous skin rashes were diagnosed as heat rashes or as the result of a fungus. The VA never really responded to the many seriously hurt veterans until they organized themselves into groups and put political pressure on the government and on Dow Chemical, Agent Orange's manufacturer. The most likely conclusion about the government's behavior is that some officials decided that admissions of responsibility for the harm caused by the herbicide would be exceptionally costly.

Another issue that incites mistrust and resentment is the POW-MIA (prisoner-of-war, missing-in-action) controversy. Approximately 2,500 POWs are unaccounted for and there were many reports of live sightings as late as the mid-1980s. Prisoners were being repatriated until the Paris peace talks broke off in 1973, when the flow of prisoners abruptly ceased. *Life* magazine summarized this issue in November 1987 (Brewster, 1987). The government's lack of official recognition of the POW issue is criticized by many veterans who see it as one more piece of proof that Vietnam veterans are abandoned by those who sent them to fight. In this case, the abandonment is not even symbolic, it is actual abandonment to captors. It is clear that Vietnam veterans are able to focus on a number of issues that seem to set them apart from the population. This separation complicated post-war adjustment and exacerbated PTSD.

Differential diagnosis of PTSD is complicated by similarities to a number of disorders, the many aforementioned social factors, and the reticence of veterans to declare their symptoms openly. To declare oneself as suffering from delayed stress is similar to stating that one is too weak for duty; there is a "taint" and one's manhood is questioned. Veterans are frequently reluctant to present their symptoms, except for those active pension seekers who have memorized the symptoms from the *DSM-III*. Further, PTSD is likely to be a complicated diagnosis. It may be associated with depression, withdrawal, substance abuse, or some disruptive behavior.

FORENSIC APPLICATION

The major forensic use of PTSD for Vietnam veterans has been as a part of the defense for veterans accused of violent crimes. Whereas civilians have used the disorder as a reason to sue offending parties, it is nearly impossible for a veteran to sue the government. In fact, a federal law passed in the post-Civil War era prohibits an attorney from receiving more than $1 for aiding a veteran in a claim against the government.

It has been noted that a legal defense based on PTSD is difficult for psychiatrists (Sparr & Atkinson, 1986), but if such a defense is necessary, it must be pursued. Legal defenses based on insanity, or diminished capacity, are complicated and difficult in any case. Convincing a judge and jury that PTSD from a war that took place 15 years earlier is related to expression of criminal behavior may be nearly impossible. The insanity defense itself has been harshly questioned since such conflicting testimony was offered in recent trials, including those of Patty Hearst and John Hinckley.

Perhaps the most dramatic phenomena associated with Vietnam veterans' adjustment are the public incidents in which veterans with weapons have barricaded themselves and taken hostages. Such incidents have been romanticized in television dramas, and have probably contributed to stigmatizing veterans. Some real events, such as the San Ysidro McDonald's tragedy and the Oklahoma City Post Office disaster, have been erroneously attributed to veterans.

Blank (1985) suggests that there have been a few hundred legal cases since 1979 where flashbacks have played some role. He cites four cases in which punishment has been mitigated because of stress disorder associated with a flashback in Vietnam veterans. Blank states that unconscious flashbacks are "sudden, discrete experience(s), leading to actions, where the manifest psychic content is only indirectly related to the war; in addition the veteran does not have conscious awareness of reliving events in Vietnam, neither at the time of the flashback, or later" (p. 297). The subject is dissociated from his behavior and should be handled carefully in the event of police confrontation. Careful management and treatment are probably best carried out by a professional who understands veterans and PTSD. One who is also a Vietnam veteran is frequently able to establish rapport when others cannot. Blank says that PTSD has gained a legal status similar to that of hysterical dissociative states, acute stress reactions, and acute psychoses. Since many attorneys will do whatever is possible to defend their clients, PTSD is likely to have been misused in the courtroom. Sparr and Atkinson (1986) cite two cases where the defense claimed PTSD as a cause for murder. Both clients lost. The prosecution was able to prove that their combat experience was minimal and not consistent with their claims of extensive combat.

Sparr and Atkinson (1986) went on to discuss PTSD as an insanity defense. Of course, any posing of mental disorder as a cause of violent crime will be intently scrutinized by the court. For a defense based on PTSD to be useful, it must be established that the accused suffers from PTSD, and that the symptoms of PTSD relate to the crime. Another way of saying it is this: The criminal behavior is so strongly related to the PTSD that the defendant's responsibility is mitigated.

Both Sparr and Atkinson (1986) and Blank (1985) stress the importance of a thorough and detailed military history for understanding PTSD in any Vietnam veteran. This history should be thorough because small details that are important to the disorder can be glossed over and missed because the subject may not wish to (or cannot) discuss the particulars. A thorough history is also important to establish the PTSD diagnosis. Finally, a thorough and detailed history may be the beginning of therapy for the veteran, who ultimately must disclose to explore the meaning of the traumatic experiences.

While PTSD is still an ephemeral phenomenon to many older mental health professionals who were trained in the analytic tradition, the diagnosis is now clearly established and is quite useful to the psychiatric community. It is perhaps most useful as a legal defense when it can be clearly linked to the crime. The difficulty of establishing PTSD as a fact in an individual's case can be attested to by many veterans who have been unable to convince the VA of any disability.

The recency of the diagnosis, its history, its association with malingering or psychoanalytically influenced ideas of predisposing neurosis and the overlap with other entities, have militated against its acceptance. Further, the social and political factors associated with the Vietnam war have inhibited investigation.

Fortunately, the work of some dedicated clinicians and scholars (e.g., Blank, 1982, 1985; Bourne, 1970; Figley, 1978, 1985; Horowitz, 1974; Sonnenberg, Blank, & Talbott, 1985) is clear and apparently unbiased. Public interest has also been aroused by the 10th anniversary parades in 1985, and by a number of recent books and movies about the Vietnam war.

Herbert J. Cross, PhD, taught in the clinical psychology program at the University of Connecticut for 7 years before joining the faculty at Pullman, Washington, where he is currently Professor of Psychology and Director of the Human Relations Center. He received his doctorate in psychology in 1965 from Syracuse University. He is a member of the Washington Board of Psychologist Examiners and Chair of the Executive Board of the Association of Directors of Psychology Training Clinics. His specialties are personality assessment, professional issues, and hypnotherapy, and he has served as a volunteer leader for a Vietnam veterans' self-help group since 1984. Dr. Cross may be contacted at the Human Relations Center, Washington State University, Pullman, WA 99165.

REFERENCES

American Psychiatric Association. (1952). *Diagnostic and Statistical Manual of Mental Disorders*. Washington, DC: Author.

American Psychiatric Association. (1968). *Diagnostic and Statistical Manual of Mental Disorders* (2nd ed.). Washington, DC: Author.

American Psychiatric Association. (1980). *Diagnostic and Statistical Manual of Mental Disorders* (3rd ed.). Washington, DC: Author.

American Psychiatric Association. (1987). *Diagnostic and Statistical Manual of Mental Disorders* (3rd ed. rev.). Washington, DC: Author.

Baritz, L. (1985). *Backfire: American Culture and the Vietnam War*. New York: Ballantine.

Blank, A. S. (1982). Stresses of war: The example of Vietnam. In L. Goldberger & S. Breznitz (Eds.), *Handbook of Stress: Theoretical and Clinical Aspects* (pp. 631-643). New York: Free Press.

Blank. A. S. (1985). The unconscious flashback to the war in Vietnam veterans: Clinical mystery, legal defense, and community problem. In S. M. Sonnenberg, A. S. Blank, & J. A. Talbott (Eds.), *The Trauma of War:*

Stress and Recovery in Vietnam Veterans (pp. 293-308). Washington, DC: American Psychiatric Press.

Boulanger, G. (1985). Post-traumatic stress disorder: An old problem with a new name. In S. M. Sonnenberg, A. S. Blank, & J. A. Talbott (Eds.), *The Trauma of War: Stress and Recovery in Vietnam Veterans* (pp. 13-29). Washington, DC: American Psychiatric Press.

Bourne, P. G. (1970). *Men, Stress and Vietnam*. Boston: Little, Brown.

Brewster, T. (1987, November). Missing. *Life*, pp. 110-124.

Cross, H. J., & Kleinhesselink, R. R. (1985). The impact of the 1960's on adolescence. *Journal of Early Adolescence, 5,* 517-532.

Erichsen, J. E. (1882). *On Concussion of the Spine: Nervous Shock and Other Obscure Injuries of the Nervous System in Their Clinical and Medico-Legal Aspects.* London: Longmans, Green & Co.

Figley, C. R. (Ed.). (1978). *Stress Disorders Among Vietnam Veterans: Theory, Research and Treatment.* New York: Brunner/Mazel.

Figley, C. R. (1985). *Trauma and Its Wake: The Study and Treatment of Post-Traumatic Stress Disorder.* New York: Brunner/Mazel.

Frankl, V. E. (1962). *Man's Search for Meaning.* New York: Simon & Schuster.

Grinker, R. R., & Spiegel, J. P. (1945). *Men Under Stress.* Philadelphia: Blakiston.

Horowitz, M. (1974). Stress response syndromes: Character style and brief psychotherapy. *Archives of General Psychiatry, 31,* 769-781.

Horowitz, M. (1986). Stress-response syndromes: A review of post-traumatic and adjustment disorder. *Hospital and Community Psychiatry, 37,* 241-249.

Jurich, A. P. (1983). The Saigon of the family's mind: Family therapy with families of Vietnam veterans. *Journal of Marital and Family Therapy, 9,* 355-363.

Kormos, H. R. (1978). The nature of combat stress. In C. R. Figley (Ed.), *Stress Disorders Among Vietnam Veterans: Theory, Research and Treatment* (pp. 3-22). New York: Brunner/Mazel.

LaBarre, W. (1954). *The Human Animal.* Chicago: University of Chicago Press.

Lazarus, R. S., & Golden, G. (1981). The function of denial in stress, coping, and aging. In E. McGaugh & S.

Kiesler (Eds.), *Biology, Behavior, and Aging* (pp. 283-304). New York: Academic Press.

Robins, L. (1981). National Institute of Mental Health diagnostic interview schedule. *Archives of General Psychiatry, 38,* 381-389.

Shatan, C. F. (1978). Stress disorders among Vietnam veterans: The emotional content of combat continues. In C. R. Figley (Ed.), *Stress Disorders Among Vietnam Veterans: Theory, Research and Treatment* (pp. 43-52). New York: Brunner/Mazel.

Sonnenberg, S. M., Blank, A. S., & Talbott, J. A. (Eds.). (1985). *Stress and Recovery in Vietnam Veterans.* Washington, DC: American Psychiatric Press.

Sparr, L. F., & Atkinson, R. M. (1986). Post-traumatic stress disorder as an insanity defense: Medicolegal quicksand. *American Journal of Psychiatry, 143,* 608-612.

Stouffer, S., Suchman, E., Devinney, L., Star, S., & Williams, R. (1949). *The American Soldier: Adjustment During Army Life.* Princeton, NJ: Princeton University Press.

Summers, H. G. (1982). *On Strategy: A Critical Analysis of the Vietnam War.* New York: Dell.

Taylor, S. E. (1983). Adjustment to threatening events: A theory of cognitive adaptation. *American Psychologist, 38,* 1161-1173.

Trimble, M. R. (1985). Post-traumatic stress disorder: History of a concept. In C. A. Figley (Ed.), *Trauma and Its Wake: The Study and Treatment of Post-Traumatic Stress Disorder* (pp. 5-14). New York: Brunner/Mazel.

Wilcox, F. A. (1983). *Waiting for an Army to Die.* New York: Vintage.

Williams, T. (1980). *Post-Traumatic Stress Disorders of Vietnam Veterans.* Cincinnati, OH: Disabled American Veterans.

5.

Reactions to Childhood Sexual Abuse: Implications for Post-Traumatic Stress Disorder

Cindy L. Miller-Perrin and Sandy K. Wurtele

CHILD SEXUAL ABUSE

Historically, professionals have had difficulty in accepting the existence of psychological and psychiatric sequelae in the child victim of disaster (Benedek, 1985). This reluctance is perhaps most notable regarding sexual abuse victims. Sigmund Freud's pronouncement that accounts of childhood sexual events represent fantasies (Masson, 1984) set in motion a firm resistance on the part of both therapists and victims to address the reality and severity of child sexual abuse. Since Freud's time there have been those at one end of the continuum who claim that childhood sexual experiences with adults can be beneficial (Guyon, 1941; J. Henderson, 1983; Yates, 1978). Others have suggested that children who are sexually exploited by adults do not suffer mental harm - either initially, or in the long term (Gagnon, 1965; Kinsey et al., 1953; Yates, 1978; Yorukoglu & Kemph, 1966). Still others have argued that child victims are harmed only later as adults (MacFarlane, 1978; Sloane & Karpinski, 1942). To explain why sexual victimization does not result in immediate harm, some have argued that since the child victim encourages, seduces, or otherwise brings on the sexual victimization, the encounter cannot be damaging (Bender & Blau, 1937; Bender & Grugett, 1952; D. J. Henderson, 1972). Others acknowledge the existence of psychological sequelae but contend that the symptoms subside relatively quickly (Yorukoglu & Kemph, 1966) or attribute them to more longstanding psychiatric problems (Bender & Grugett, 1952).

The first part of the chapter will address the question, "Can child sexual victimization result in harmful effects?" We will first review the literature on the initial and long-term effects of sexual abuse, organizing the most substantiated findings into categories that lend support to the existence of a specific symptom complex. Next, this sexual abuse trauma syndrome will be compared with post-traumatic stress disorder (PTSD) in an attempt to answer the question, "Can the *Diagnostic and Statistical Manual of Mental Disorders* (*DSM-III-R*, American Psychiatric Association, 1987) criteria for post-traumatic stress disorder, as validated for adults, be directly applied to children who have been sexually abused?" We will also examine the evidence as to whether a PTSD diagnosis may be appropriate for adults who present symptoms associated with childhood sexual trauma. Finally, we will discuss the research and clinical implications of sexual-abuse-related PTSD.

CAN CHILD SEXUAL VICTIMIZATION RESULT IN HARMFUL EFFECTS?

To answer this question, four different types of sample populations have been studied: (a) children and adolescents who have been recently abused, (b) college students abused as children, (c) adults seeking treatment who were abused as children, and (d) random populations of college students and adults abused as children. Findings obtained from children and adolescents soon after the abuse have been used to establish initial effects whereas long-term effects have been studied using college students and adults abused as children.

Research efforts in this area have been plagued by serious methodological problems. For example, the definition of "sexual abuse" varies across studies (Browne & Finkelhor, 1986; D. S. Everstine & L. Everstine, 1983; P. B. Mrazek, 1983). In addition, important characteristics of the abusive situation (e.g., extent of sexual contact, affective nature of the relationship to the perpetrator, age at the onset of abuse, duration and frequency of abuse, etc.) are often ignored despite the fact that they may determine the impact of sexual abuse (Browne & Finkelhor, 1986; D. S. Everstine & L. Everstine, 1983; Lusk & Waterman, 1986). Many studies utilize single- or multiple-case reports. While these studies provide valuable information about the complex and diverse nature of sexually abusive experiences and help to generate hypotheses, they do not permit the establishment of general principles (P. B. Mrazek, 1983). Several studies have failed to include control or contrast groups (D. S. Everstine & L. Everstine, 1983; P. B. Mrazek, 1983), and others employed subjective, unstandardized interviews and assessment devices (Browne & Finkelhor, 1986; P. B. Mrazek & D. A. Mrazek, 1981). Studies utilizing adult and college student samples are retrospective in nature; they present information that is susceptible to a great deal of distortion. In addition, college student populations are biased in terms of intelligence, social class, and motivation (P. B. Mrazek, 1983). Finally, studying the effects of adolescents or adults abused as children precludes the establishment of cause-and-effect relationships (P. B. Mrazek, 1983). In the absence of longitudinal studies, we are unable to determine whether the associations between early sexual abuse and later consequences are indeed causally related.

In short, advancements in determining the effects of sexual abuse have been limited by the methodological weaknesses of the studies. Furthermore, there is an extraordinary amount of variability in the effects described in the literature (MacFarlane & Waterman, 1986; Nakashima & Zakus, 1979; J. J. Peters, 1974). Undoubtedly there is a relationship between the variability in findings and methodological weaknesses of the studies. Despite the lack of methodological rigor and diverse findings, however, several similarities across samples can be noted. In this section, symptom pictures for sexually abused children and adolescents and adults abused as children will be reviewed.

INITIAL EFFECTS

P. B. Mrazek and D. A. Mrazek (1981) have summarized initial effects of sexual abuse based on reports appearing in the literature since the 1930s. Their information on the immediate effects of sexual abuse is derived primarily from clinical case material such as single-case studies, composite accounts of multiple patients, and chart reviews. In contrast, Browne and Finkelhor (1986) have focused only on "empirical" studies, which they define as "any research that attempted to quantify the extent to which a sequelae to sexual abuse appeared in a specific population" (p. 66). These latter researchers concluded that the empirical literature on the effects of child sexual abuse supports many of the initial effects reported in the clinical literature. The specific immediate effects of childhood sexual abuse (i.e., those reactions occurring within 2 years of the termination of abuse) have been categorized into the six general areas presented in Table 5.1 (pp. 95-96). These areas include affective, physical, social functioning, cognitive, sexuality, and antisocial or acting-out effects.

Clinical Studies. In general, clinical studies have attempted only to describe the symptom picture of child and adolescent victims. Affective effects include (a) anxiety manifested as fears and phobias (Mian et al., 1986; Tilelli, Tarek, & Jaffe, 1980), anxiety states (Bender & Blau, 1937), nightmares (Mian et al., 1986; Tilelli et al., 1980), recurring dreams (Burgess & Holmstrom, 1975), nail biting (Burton, 1968), clinging behavior (Mian et al., 1986), somatization (Dixon, Arnold, & Calestro, 1978; Lewis & Sarrell, 1969; Maisch, 1972; Tilelli et al., 1980), and separation anxiety (Brandt & Tisza, 1977); (b) depression manifested as pessimism and suicidal ideation (Bender & Blau, 1937; Ferenczi, 1949; Forbes, 1972; Kaufman, Peck, & Tagiuri, 1954; Maisch, 1972; Mehta et al., 1979; Nakashima & Zakus, 1977), loss of self-esteem (DeFrancis, 1969), and guilt and shame (DeFrancis, 1969; Rosenfeld, Nadelson, & Krieger, 1979); and (c) anger and hostility manifested as tantrums (Adams-Tucker, 1981), arguing with peers (Burgess, Groth, & McCausland, 1981), and irritability (Burgess et al., 1984).

Physical effects include sleep difficulties (Burgess et al., 1981), venereal disease (Branch & Paxton, 1965), pregnancy (Mehta et al., 1979), and impulsive, self-damaging behavior (Dixon et al., 1978). Social functioning effects include increased affection-seeking behavior (Burton, 1968), bewilderment concerning social relations (Bender & Blau, 1937), withdrawal (Adams-Tucker, 1981; Bender & Blau, 1937; Burgess et al., 1981), and poor peer relationships (Riggs, 1982). Among cognitive effects are learning difficulties (Kaufman et al., 1954; Rosenfeld et al., 1979), declining grades (Burgess et al., 1981), the use of dissociation (Adams-Tucker, 1985; Nielson, 1983), and problems concentrating on tasks because of short attention spans (Shaw & Meier, 1983). Antisocial or acting-out

TABLE 5.1: INITIAL EFFECTS REPORTED AMONG SEXUALLY ABUSED CHILDREN AND ADOLESCENTS

Type of Effect	Specific Problem	Specific Symptoms
Affective	Depression	Pessimism, suicidal ideation, sadness, feelings of guilt and shame, low self-esteem
	Anxiety	Fears (especially of adults) and phobias, recurring dreams, nightmares, somatic symptoms (headache, stomach problems), nail biting, clinging behavior, separation anxiety, flashbacks
	Hostility or Anger	Irritability, tantrums, quarreling
Physical		Sleep difficulties, changes in appetite, pregnancy
Social Functioning		Increased affection seeking, early marriages by adolescent victims, bewilderment concerning social relations, withdrawal, poor peer relationships
Cognitive	Learning Difficulties	Inability to concentrate, short attention span, deterioration of academic performance, dissociation

Type of Effect	Specific Problem	Specific Symptoms
Antisocial Behavior or Acting Out		Prostitution, promiscuity, delinquency, stealing, impulsivity, truancy, dropping out of school, substance abuse, running away
Sexuality	Sexual Adjustment	Open masturbation, excessive sexual curiosity, frequent exposure of genitals, acting-out sexual delinquency, molestation of younger children

effects include behavior problems and delinquency (Maisch, 1972; Nakashima & Zakus, 1977), promiscuity (Lukianowicz, 1972; Maisch, 1972; Sloane & Karpinski, 1942), stealing (Weiss et al., 1955), running away from home (Browning & Boatman, 1977; Kaufman et al., 1954), and substance abuse (Herman & Hirschman, 1981; Riggs, 1972; Summit, 1983). Sexuality effects are such effects as open masturbation (Isaacs, 1933), excessive sexual curiosity (Bender & Blau, 1937), sudden rush into heterosexual activities (Herman & Hirschman, 1981), and acting-out sexual delinquency, seemingly purposeless and not enjoyed (Kaufman et al., 1954; Rabinovitch, 1953).

Empirical Studies. The most common initial effect noted in the empirical literature, similar to reports in the clinical literature, is fear (Browne & Finkelhor, 1986). The proportions of victims presenting with fear-related symptoms vary, but all studies report substantially high percentages: 83% in DeFrancis (1969), 40% in Anderson, Bach, and Griffith (1981), and 45% of the 7- to 13-year-olds in Tufts (1984). In addition, Mannarino and Cohen (1986) recently found several anxiety-related symptoms in their sample of 45 sexually abused children referred by a local child welfare agency including: nightmares (56%), anxiety (22%), and clinging behavior (22%). Other reports have indicated the presence of nightmares (J. J. Peters, 1976) and anxiety states (Meiselman, 1978). Anxiety manifested as somatic complaints is also well documented. For example, Mannarino and Cohen (1986) found enuresis to be a problem for 18% of their sample. In addition, Adams-Tucker (1982) noted clinically significant psychosomatic problems as a result of sexual victimization.

Another initial affective effect cited in the clinical literature and confirmed in the empirical literature is the reaction of anger or hostility. Adams-Tucker (1982) found the abused children in her sample to exhibit a high degree of oppositional difficulty with parents, siblings, and peers as well as aggressive behaviors as indicated on the Louisville Behavior Checklist (LBC; Miller, 1981). Tufts' (1984) researchers found that 45%-50% of latency (7- to 13-year-olds) and 13%-17% of preschool children (4- to 6-year-olds) showed substantially elevated scores on measures of aggression and antisocial behavior on the LBC. In addition, scores were elevated on a measure of hostility directed outward: preschool (25%), latency (35%), and adolescent (23%). DeFrancis (1969) also found that 55% of his sample manifested behavioral disturbances such as active defiance, disruptive behavior within the family, and quarreling and fighting with siblings or classmates.

Depression is another affective effect of childhood sexual abuse indicated in the empirical literature. Anderson et al. (1981) found that 25% of their sample was depressed. Mannarino and Cohen (1986) found sadness in 22% of their sample rated by parents and evaluators on a symptom checklist. In addition, lowered self-esteem was also documented in 58% of DeFrancis' (1969) sample. However, Tufts' (1984) researchers, using the Purdue Self-Concept Scale, did not find lower self-esteem among sexually abused children compared with a normal population of children. Guilt and shame are other frequently observed reactions in both the clinical and empirical literature. DeFrancis (1969) found that 64% of his sample expressed guilt while Anderson et al. (1981) reported guilt reactions in 25% of the victims.

The physical effects observed in the clinical literature are also frequently cited in the empirical literature. Anderson et al. (1981) and J. J. Peters (1976) found that 17% and 31%, respectively, of their samples of sexually abused children had difficulty sleeping. In addition, 5%-7% (Anderson et al., 1981) and 20% (J. J. Peters, 1976) of

97

victims showed changes in eating habits. Adolescent pregnancy is another physical complication: DeFrancis (1969) found 11% of the child victims became pregnant as a result of their abuse.

Social functioning effects have been documented in several studies and include withdrawal (Adams-Tucker, 1982), early marriages by adolescent victims (Meiselman, 1978), and poor peer relations (Lusk & Waterman, 1986). Antisocial or acting-out effects have also been observed in several studies. Two studies found high percentages of running away among their samples: 33% (Herman, 1981) and 50% (Meiselman, 1978). J. J. Peters (1976) also noted that 10% of his sample dropped out of school before age 12. Additionally, 20% of the Anderson et al. (1981) sample had problems of truancy.

Finally, as the clinical literature has suggested, there are sexuality effects that the empirical literature generally supports. For example, inappropriate sexual behavior (including open masturbation, excessive sexual curiosity, and frequent exposure of genitals) was found in 33% of the sexually abused children in the Tufts' study (1984). Mannarino and Cohen (1986) noted inappropriate sexual behavior in 16% of their sample. Friedrich, Urquiza, and Beilke (1986) distinguished between inappropriate sexual behavior in male and female children and found that 70% of the boys and 44% of the girls had elevated scores on the sexual problems scale of the Child Behavior Checklist (Achenbach & Edelbrock, 1983). Two-thirds of the 125 children presenting at an acute-care hospital because of sexual abuse had physical or behavioral symptoms, and almost a fifth of them showed inappropriate sexual behavior such as seductive behavior and requests for sexual stimulation (Mian et al., 1986).

Child sexual abuse has been associated with a range of psychopathology (Lusk & Waterman, 1986). For example, DeFrancis (1969) reported that 66% of the victims in his sample were emotionally disturbed by the molestation (52% mildly to moderately, 14% seriously). Only 24% were judged to be emotionally stable after the abuse. Adams-Tucker (1982) studied 28 sexually abused children referred for treatment and found psychopathology in the "moderate to severe" range among most victims. While these problems were more severe than those of the typical outpatient children at her clinic, they were judged to be less severe than those of the average inpatient. Mannarino and Cohen (1986) found that of 45 sexually abused children studied, 69% had clinically significant psychological symptoms on a Likert-type symptom checklist while 31% had minor or no symptoms. Anderson et al. (1981) reviewed clinical charts of 155 female adolescent sexual assault victims who had received treatment and reported psychosocial complications in 63% of them. "Internalized" psychosocial complications (e.g., sleep and eating disturbances, fears and phobias, depression, guilt, shame, and anger) were observed in 49%-67% of female victims and "externalized" sequelae (e.g., school problems and running away) were noted in 21%-66% of the victims. Researchers at the Tufts' New England Medical Center (Tufts, 1984) gathered data on children who had been victimized or revealed their victimization within the previous 6 months. Seventeen percent of the preschool group (4-6 years) met the criteria for "clinically significant pathology," 40% of the latency age group (7-13 years) scored in the seriously disturbed range, while few of the adolescent victims (14-18 years) exhibited severe psychopathology.

Recently, Gomes-Schwartz, Horowitz, and Sauzier (1985) evaluated 112 children who had been sexually victimized or revealed their victimization within the 6 months preceding referral. Findings indicated that both the preschool (4-6 years) and school-age groups (7-13 years) exhibited significantly more overall behavioral disturbances than children of comparable ages in the general population, while relatively small proportions of adolescents (14-18 years) exhibited severe pathology. All three groups exhibited less overall pathology and fewer specific difficulties than children of comparable ages receiving psychiatric services. Friedrich et al. (1986) also found a differential impact of sexual abuse for different ages of female children. Results indicated that on a measure of overall disturbance (the Child Behavior Checklist; Achenbach & Edelbrock, 1983), younger children (up to age 5) demonstrated a tendency to score high on the Internalizing Scale (including fearful, inhibited, depressed, and overcontrolled behaviors) whereas older children (6-12 years) were more likely to have elevated scores on the Externalizing Scale (aggressive, antisocial, and undercontrolled behaviors). Overall, 46% of subjects had significantly elevated scores on the Internalizing Scale and 39% had elevated scores on the Externalizing Scale.

In contrast to earlier reports suggesting that sexual encounters between adults and children may have no harmful effects, more recent empirical and clinical findings indicate that some portion of the sexual abuse victim population is severely affected by sexual abuse and manifests symptom-specific trauma. In their review of the literature, Browne and Finkelhor (1986) concluded that from 20% to 40% of abused children seen by clinicians manifest pathological disturbance. Taken alone, this range is alarming in itself and supports a definite affirmative response to our question, "Can child sexual victimization result in [initial] harmful effects?" When one considers that these figures are based on victims who were discovered or disclosed their abuse and were receiving treatment, it becomes possible to speculate that the range may extend even higher if all victims were studied. Assuming that discovery or disclosure terminates the abuse, this protection may reduce the severity of abuse-related sequelae. For those victimized children and adolescents who are not discovered or do not disclose, the traumatogenic effects continue unabated, and remain undocumented.

LONG-TERM EFFECTS

The possible long-term effects of child sexual abuse have been summarized and reviewed (Browne & Finkelhor, 1986; P. B. Mrazek & D. A. Mrazek, 1981) and appear to be remarkably similar to the initial effects (P. B. Mrazek, 1983). Long-term effects have been studied using clinical and random samples of adults and college women. In general, consistent symptom pictures have been described across all sample populations. The long-term effects of childhood sexual abuse are categorized in Table 5.2 (pp. 101-102) and will be reviewed according to the type of sample investigated.

Clinical Samples. In the affective realm, depression is the symptom most commonly reported among adults abused as children (Browne & Finkelhor, 1986; Courtois & Watts, 1982). For example, Meiselman (1978) reported depressive symptoms in 35% of incest victims compared with 23% of the comparison group. In addition, Herman (1981) noted major depressive symptoms in 60% of the incest victims in her study although 55% of the comparison group also reported depression. Adults sexually abused as children also show self-destructive behavior such as suicide and suicidal ideation (Briere, 1984; Briere

TABLE 5.2: LONG-TERM EFFECTS REPORTED AMONG ADULTS SEXUALLY ABUSED AS CHILDREN

Type of Effect	Specific Problem	Specific Symptoms
Affective	Depression	Suicide, suicidal ideation, desire to hurt self, poor self-image, low self-esteem, dysphoric affect, feelings of guilt
	Anxiety	Tension, anxiety attacks, nightmares, somatic symptoms (migraine, stomach problems, aches and pains, skin disorders), fear of men, flashbacks, recurring nightmares, phobic behavior
Physical		Sleep difficulties, obesity, eating disorders
Social Functioning		Feelings of isolation and alienation, social isolation, difficulty establishing close human relationships, problems parenting
Cognitive		Inability to concentrate, intrusive, repetitive thoughts, dissociation, amnesia
Antisocial Behavior or Acting Out		Prostitution, promiscuity, substance abuse

101

Type of Effect	Specific Problem	Specific Symptoms
Sexuality	Sexual Adjustment	Sexual anxiety, sexual guilt, dissatisfaction with sexual relationships, anorgasmia, less sexual responsivity, avoidance of men and sexual activity

& Runtz, 1986; Harrison, Lumry, & Claypatch, 1984; Herman, 1981; Rhinehart, 1961), and a desire to hurt themselves (Briere, 1984). In addition, feelings of guilt, poor self-image, and low self-esteem among this population have been repeatedly reported (Herman, 1981; Meiselman, 1978; Sloane & Karpinski, 1942; Tsai & Wagner, 1978).

Another reaction observed in adults molested as children is elevated anxiety. Symptoms include anxiety attacks (Briere, 1984), nightmares (Briere, 1984; Meiselman, 1978), somatic symptoms (most often migraine, as well as stomach ailments, disabling aches and pains, and skin disorders; Forward & Buck, 1978), flashbacks and recurring nightmares of the incident (Donaldson & Gardner, 1985; Meiselman, 1978), and fear of men in addition to other phobic behavior (Briere, 1984; Courtois & Watts, 1982; Meiselman, 1978).

Physical effects documented in the literature include difficulty sleeping (Briere, 1984), obesity (Meiselman, 1978), and eating disorders (Oppenheimer, Palmer, & Brandon, 1984). In a British eating disorders treatment program, 34% of the participants reported having been sexually abused before the age of 15 (Oppenheimer et al., 1984). These researchers have suggested that eating disorders may be a more common long-term effect of childhood sexual victimization than is currently recognized.

In the social and interpersonal realm, victimized adults often report feeling isolated and alienated (Briere, 1984; Herman, 1981; Tsai & Wagner, 1978), and have difficulty establishing close human relationships (Steele & Alexander, 1981; Tsai & Wagner, 1978). Evidence is also accumulating to suggest that childhood sexual abuse affects later parenting. Goodwin, McCarthy, and DiVasto (1981) found that 24% of the mothers in their sample of child-abusing families reported having been sexually victimized as children, compared with 3% of mothers in a nonabusive control group. Women who have been victimized as children also appear to be vulnerable to revictimization later in life. In her random sample of 930 women, Russell (1986) found that 33%-68% of the sexual abuse victims (the percentages varied depending on the seriousness of the abuse) were subsequently raped, compared with 17% of women who were not victimized as children. Women abused as children were also more likely to be abused by their husbands. Russell found that 38%-48% of her sample had physically violent husbands compared with 17% of nonvictimized women. Similarly, Briere (1984) found that 49% of his clinical sexual abuse sample had been battered in adult relationships compared with 18% of a nonvictim group.

Effects on cognitive functioning have also been reported and include an inability to concentrate (Courtois & Watts, 1982), an unintegrated sense of identity (Katan, 1973; Steele & Alexander, 1981), and intrusive, repetitious thoughts (Donaldson & Gardner, 1985; Silver, Boon, & Stones, 1983). Regarding dissociative effects, several researchers have drawn attention to the issue of dissociation as a long-term effect of childhood sexual abuse. Briere and Runtz (1985) found that sexual abuse victims in a clinical setting reported more symptoms of dissociation and "spaciness" (42% versus 22% for controls), as well as "out of body experiences" (21% versus 8%) and feeling that things are unreal (33% versus 11%). These researchers have hypothesized that dissociation is a strategy that victims use to escape from the unpleasant abuse experience and that later this becomes an autonomous symptom. Others have described dissociative phenomena in the sexually abused adults they studied (e.g., Courtois & Watts, 1982; Lindberg & Distad, 1985) as well as varying degrees of amnesia (Herman & Schatzow, 1987). Evidence for sexual abuse in the history of multiple personality disorder cases is also accumulating (e.g., Fagan & McMahon, 1984; Kluft, 1984; Sachs, Goodwin, & Braun, in press). For example, in his review of multiple personality disorder cases published in the literature, Putnam (1984) found that a history of childhood sexual abuse was reported in 70% of the patients.

An association between child sexual abuse and later substance abuse has also been noted. For example, Herman (1981) found that 35% of the women with incestuous fathers in her clinical sample abused drugs and alcohol (versus 5% of the women with seductive but not incestuous fathers). Similarly, Briere (1984) found that 27% of the childhood sexual abuse victims seen at a community mental health center had a history of alcoholism (versus 11% of nonvictims) and 21% had a history of drug addiction (versus 2% of the nonvictims). Kovach (1983) studied 117 women who were members of Alcoholics Anonymous and found almost 30% had experienced incest during their childhoods.

Almost all clinical studies document problems in victimized women related to sexual adjustment (Briere, 1984; Browne & Finkelhor, 1986; Herman, 1981; Langmade, 1983; Meiselman, 1978). These problems include sexual anxiety, sexual guilt, dissatisfaction with sexual relationships (Langmade, 1983; Van Buskirk & Cole, 1983), later avoidance of men and sexual activity (Meiselman, 1978; Tsai & Wagner, 1978), prostitution (James & Meyerding, 1977; Silbert & Pines, 1981), promiscuity (de Young, 1982; Herman, 1981; Meiselman, 1978), and difficulties in achieving orgasm and being sexually responsive (Tsai, Feldman-Summers, & Edgar, 1979).

Random Samples. Data from several random community samples have buttressed clinical findings. For example, results from two random samples of women found that subjects with a history of sexual abuse were more depressed than nonabused women (Bagley & Ramsay, 1985; S. D. Peters, 1984), had a greater number of depressive episodes over time, and were more likely to be hospitalized for depression than nonvictims (S. D. Peters, 1984). In addition, community studies have affirmed an association between childhood sexual abuse and suicidal ideation or deliberate attempts at self-harm (Bagley & Ramsay, 1985). Random samples have also supported the finding of anxiety and tension among adults abused as children (Bagley & Ramsay, 1985), along with negative self-concept (Bagley & Ramsay, 1985; Courtois, 1979), sexual adjustment problems (Courtois, 1979), promiscuity (Courtois, 1979), and isolation and alienation (Courtois, 1979).

College Populations. Findings obtained from studies of college students parallel those from clinical samples. For example, Sedney and Brooks (1984) and Briere and Runtz (1985) found a greater likelihood for sexually

abused students to report symptoms of depression compared with a control group. In addition, victimized college samples have reported having thoughts of hurting
themselves and attempting suicide, along with such other
symptoms as nervousness and anxiety, extreme tension,
and trouble sleeping (Sedney & Brooks, 1984), phobic
anxiety (Fromuth, 1986), and sexual adjustment problems
(Finkelhor, 1979; Fromuth, 1986)

Summary. The findings of these long-term studies
indicate that many adults who experienced sexual abuse
as children have identifiable degrees of impairment as
reported in both the clinical and empirical literature. In
terms of self-assessment, 53% of intrafamilial sexual
abuse victims in Russell's (1986) community survey reported that the experience resulted in "some" or "great"
long-term effects on their lives. Finkelhor (1979) and
Courtois (1980) found that 66% and 80%, respectively, of
their adult women samples indicated that the impact of
the sexual experience was severe. Meiselman (1978) also
noted that the abused women in her sample complained of
greater severity of symptoms compared with a control
group. More specifically, 32% of the abused group were
judged to be "severely disturbed" compared with 20% of
the control group.

Thus, it is apparent that the trauma-related symptoms
exhibited by sexually abused children, adolescents, and
adults are quite similar. In addition, the evidence accumulated to date strongly suggests that childhood sexual abuse
results in very disturbing psychological sequelae in a
significant portion of its victims. The abuse experience
can affect the victim's functioning in a number of areas,
including the affective (i.e., anxiety, depression, hostility,
and anger), physical, social, cognitive, behavioral, and
sexuality realms. We will now attempt to determine
whether the symptoms of this sexual abuse trauma syndrome are similar to the symptom complex referred to as
post-traumatic stress disorder (PTSD).

STUDIES SUGGESTING A RELATIONSHIP
BETWEEN CHILDHOOD SEXUAL TRAUMA
AND POST-TRAUMATIC STRESS DISORDER

In the American Psychiatric Association's (1987)
revised third edition of the *Diagnostic and Statistical*

Manual of Mental Disorders (*DSM-III-R*), PTSD is defined as follows:

> The essential feature of this disorder is the development of characteristic symptoms following a psychologically distressing event that is outside the range of usual human experience (i.e., outside the range of such common experiences as simple bereavement, chronic illness, business losses, and marital conflict). The stressor producing this syndrome would be markedly distressing to almost anyone, and is usually experienced with intense fear, terror, and helplessness. The characteristic symptoms involve reexperiencing the traumatic event, avoidance of stimuli associated with the event or numbing of general responsiveness, and increased arousal. The diagnosis is not made if the disturbance lasts less than one month. (p. 247)

Some of the associated features described in the *DSM-III-R* are symptoms of depression and anxiety, impulsive behavior, or such symptoms as failing memory, difficulty concentrating, emotional lability, headache, vertigo, and painful guilt feelings. Age-specific features of PTSD include repetitive play in young children as a form of reliving the trauma. Occasionally, children may refuse to discuss the trauma, may experience distressing dreams or a change in orientation toward the future, and may exhibit constricted affect or various physical symptoms (e.g., stomachaches or headaches). According to *DSM-III-R*, diminished responsiveness usually begins soon after the traumatic event. Re-experiencing symptoms may develop after a latency period of months or years (though avoidance symptoms have usually been present during this latency period).

In general, the phenomenon of PTSD, with a few notable exceptions, has not been widely studied among children. Post-traumatic stress disorder has been documented in children who have been kidnapped (Senior, Gladstone, & Nurcombe, 1982; Terr, 1979), victims of a slag avalanche and flooding (Lacey, 1972; Newman, 1976), exposed to homicide of a parent (Eth & Pynoos, 1985), or bitten by a dog (Gislason & Call, 1982). Part of the reason why child sexual abuse has not been regularly associated with PTSD may be the strict criteria often employed for childhood trauma. In her working definition of "trauma," Terr (1985) stated, "Psychic trauma is that emotional condition following from a sudden, unexpected, and intense external blow that overwhelmed crucial coping and defensive operations, temporarily rendering the individual helpless . . ." (p. 816). She further stated, "Some horrible, externally generated, chronic conditions in childhood--child abuse, incest, maternal deprivation--would thus be somewhat removed from the more purely 'traumatized' group because of the chronicity and lack of surprise within these ugly realities" (p. 816). Rather than being exposed to a single, unexpected incident, most child sexual abuse victims (like combat veterans) have experienced multiple assaults on the self.

In contrast to Terr's (1985) narrow definition of trauma, we have found Kluft's (1984) definition to be a more heuristic one. By analyzing the characteristics of experiences that triggered dissociative responses, he generated the following criteria for a traumatic incident: (a) the child fears for his or her own life; (b) the child fears that an important attachment figure will die; (c) the child's physical intactness or clarity of consciousness is breached or impaired; (d) the child is isolated with these fears; and (e) the child is systematically misinformed, or "brainwashed," about his or her situation. We agree with Goodwin (1985) that this pragmatic definition of trauma will better predict many of the factors associated with poor prognosis in incest victims.

POST-TRAUMATIC STRESS DISORDER IN YOUNG SEXUAL ABUSE VICTIMS

Few studies have linked the effects of childhood sexual abuse with PTSD. Burgess and her colleagues (1984) studied 66 children and adolescents who had been exploited through sex rings and pornography shows. Using a semistructured interview procedure, these researchers found differential response patterns before and after disclosure. Symptoms at post-disclosure were specifically defined as a post-traumatic stress response. Sixty-eight percent of the children reported re-experiencing the event through intrusive thoughts and flashbacks. In addition, children reported feeling nervous when certain things reminded them of the event. Vivid memories and dreams along with night terrors occurred. Sixty-two percent of the children showed diminished responsiveness to others and the environment as evidenced by reduced involvement in daily activities, withdrawal from friends and school activities, and refusal to attend school. Seventy-four percent of the children showed symptoms of excessive autonomic arousal, especially hyperalertness. In addition, the children reported that they lost their tempers easily and disliked "being startled." There were also signs of sleep disturbance, irritability, feelings of guilt, and difficulty concentrating.

In child sex rings we see many of the characteristics of trauma as defined by Kluft (1984). Many children fear for their lives (e.g., in Burgess et al., 1984, some children had vivid dreams where the offender would return and retaliate or carry out the threats made during the child's participation in the ring). Children develop strong attachments to the offender, who occupies a position of authority and familiarity to them. Thus, the child has strong ambivalent feelings - both devotion to and fear of the offender. Developmentally immature children would have difficulty making sense out of these conflicting feelings. These children are also prematurely initiated into sexual activity; some are provided with drugs and alcohol to encourage their participation. The offenders use threats of retaliation, extortion, and peer pressure to insure the secrecy of the ring and its activities, and ultimately its continuance (Burgess et al., 1981). Finally, through the grooming process children are systematically "brainwashed" into believing the activity is acceptable.

As the characteristics of ongoing, individual sexual relationships between adults and children likewise make for potentially traumatic experiences, clinicians are urged to consider making a diagnosis of PTSD. In our earlier review of the initial effects of sexual abuse, it would appear that many child victims are manifesting the signs and symptoms of PTSD. In Table 5.3 (pp. 109-111), we have identified the PTSD symptoms that have been reported among sexually abused children. By definition, all victims of repeated sexual abuse would meet criterion A (experiencing an event outside the normal range of human experience). Regarding criterion B (re-experiencing the trauma), many child victims report experiencing flashbacks, recurrent dreams, or feeling as if the traumatic event were reoccurring. Although not included as an example, we encourage clinicians to view sexual and physical acting out as indicative of such re-experiencing. Examples would include excessive masturbation, sexual

---

TABLE 5.3: CLASSIFICATION OF THE INITIAL (I) AND LONG-TERM (LT) EFFECTS OF SEXUAL ABUSE ACCORDING TO POST-TRAUMATIC STRESS DISORDER CRITERIA AND ASSOCIATED SYMPTOMS*

Diagnostic Criteria for PTSD

I;LT   A.   The person has experienced an event that is outside the range of usual human experience and that would be markedly distressing to almost anyone. (Repeated sexual abuse is used as an example of an extreme psychosocial stressor for Axis IV.)

I;LT   B.   The traumatic event is persistently re-experienced in at least one of the following ways:

       1.   Recurrent and intrusive distressing recollections of the event (e.g., in young children, repetitive play in which themes or aspects of the trauma are expressed, sexualized activity, aggressive antisocial behaviors).

I;LT   2.   Recurrent distressing dreams of the event (e.g., nightmares, recurring dreams).

I;LT   3.   Sudden acting or feeling as if the traumatic event were reoccurring (includes a sense of reliving the experience, illusions, hallucinations, and dissociative [flashback] episodes, even those that occur upon awakening or when intoxicated; e.g., flashbacks).

I;LT   4.   Intense psychological distress at exposure to events that symbolize or resemble an aspect of the traumatic event, including anniversaries of the trauma (e.g., in children, fears - especially of adults; in adults, fears of men or sexual activities).

I;LT   C.   Persistent avoidance of stimuli associated with the trauma or numbing of general responsiveness (not present before the trauma), as indicated by at least three of the following:

I;LT   1.   Efforts to avoid thoughts or feelings associated with the trauma (e.g., dissociation).

Diagnostic Criteria for PTSD

I;LT   2. Efforts to avoid activities or situations that arouse
            recollections of the trauma (e.g., phobias, refusing
            to leave home, avoidance of men).

LT   3. Inability to recall an important aspect of the trauma
            (psychogenic amnesia).

I;LT   4. Markedly diminished interest in significant activities
            (e.g., in young children, loss of recently acquired
            developmental skills such as toilet training or lan-
            guage skills, withdrawal from activities of normal
            childhood, enuresis, encopresis; in adults, social
            isolation, disinterest in sex).

I;LT   5. Feeling of detachment or estrangement from others
            (e.g., poor peer relationships, feelings of isolation
            and alienation, difficulty establishing close human
            relationships).

I;LT   6. Restricted range of affect (e.g., unable to have love
            feelings or depression).

        7. Sense of a foreshortened future (e.g., does not expect
            to have a career, marriage, children, or long life).

I;LT D. Persistent symptoms of increased arousal (not present be-
          fore the trauma), as indicated by at least two of the
          following:

I;LT   1. Difficulty falling or staying asleep (e.g., difficul-
            ties with sleep patterns).

        2. Irritability or outbursts of anger (e.g., anger and
            hostility, tantrums, opposition with parents,
            siblings, peers).

I;LT   3. Difficulty concentrating (e.g., problems in concen-
            trating/short attention span).

        4. Hypervigilance.

110

Diagnostic Criteria for PTSD

---

    5. Exaggerated startle response.

LT   6. Physiologic reactivity upon exposure to events that
            symbolize or resemble an aspect of the traumatic event
            (e.g., anxiety attacks).

Associated Features of PTSD

I;LT   A. Symptoms of depression (e.g., pessimism, suicidal idea-
            tion, loss of self-esteem, sadness, desire to hurt self).

I;LT   B. Symptoms of anxiety (e.g., in children, nail biting,
            clinging behavior, separation anxiety, somatization; in
            adults, tension, anxiety, somatization).

I;LT   C. Guilt feelings (e.g., feelings of guilt and shame).

I;LT   D. Impulsive behavior (e.g., in children, running away,
            stealing, truancy; in adults, promiscuity).

I;LT   E. Headache (e.g., in children, increased incidence of head-
            ache; in adults, increased incidence of migraine).

I;LT   F. Stomachache (e.g., increased incidence of stomachache).

        G. Emotional lability.

        H. Vertigo.

---

*Note. From Diagnostic and Statistical Manual of Mental Disorders
(3rd ed. rev., pp. 249-250) by American Psychiatric Association,
1987, Washington, DC: American Psychiatric Association. Reprinted
with permission from the American Psychiatric Association.

---

acting out, and aggressive antisocial behaviors. In this response pattern, the child masters the anxiety generated by the abuse by exploiting others. A similar pattern of endless repetition of post-traumatic play and re-enactment has been observed by Terr (1981a, 1983) in her studies of kidnapped victims. The repeated sexual acting out among abuse victims can also be viewed from a social learning theory perspective as these victims have observed the offenders exhibiting sexually victimizing behaviors, and the children have also been rewarded for participating in sexual activities.

Regarding criterion C (persistent avoidance of stimuli associated with the trauma or numbing of responsiveness), many victims exhibit avoidance of stimuli associated with the trauma through dissociative defenses. Numbing of general responsiveness is evidenced by depressive symptomatology, withdrawal from normal childhood experiences, or poor peer relationships. Many victims also exhibit the increased arousal symptoms listed in criterion D, including sleep difficulties, outbursts of anger (e.g., tantrums), and problems concentrating. Associated features noted in victims include symptoms of depression, anxiety, impulsive behavior, stomachache and headache, and guilt feelings.

In summary, sexual abuse of children is a traumatic event that, for many, results in symptoms similar to those exhibited by victims of post-traumatic stress disorder. Although researchers and clinicians have documented the existence of these individual symptoms in abuse victims, we encourage them to view these symptoms as part of the sexual abuse trauma syndrome and to consider whether the victims meet the diagnostic criteria for PTSD. A comparison of the *DSM-III-R* diagnostic criteria for PTSD and the symptoms most frequently experienced by sexual abuse victims strongly suggests that sexual-abuse-related PTSD comprises an identifiable constellation of symptoms. Psychologists must overcome their reluctance to accept the existence of psychological sequelae in the child victim of trauma (Benedek, 1985) so that psychological assistance can be immediately and appropriately provided.

POST-TRAUMATIC STRESS DISORDER IN ADULTS ABUSED AS CHILDREN

In reviewing the literature on the long-term effects of sexual abuse in women seeking therapy, Gelinas (1983) argued that the range of symptoms and problems seen in former incest victims and described in the incest literature can be accounted for, in part, by an underlying persisting negative effect that, over time and with lack of treatment, elaborates and increasingly intrudes upon the lives of the victims. Gelinas called this underlying, persistent negative effect "chronic traumatic neurosis" - now referred to as PTSD. Gelinas pointed out that neither analysts nor incest specialists have identified PTSD as a specific consequence of sexual abuse, although the clinical picture is unmistakable and there can be little doubt that former incest victims show underlying PTSD.

We have been able to locate only three studies that have recognized an association between PTSD and the effects of sexual abuse utilizing adult populations of women who were abused as children. In 1983, Kovach studied 117 women who were members of Alcoholics Anonymous in an attempt to investigate the relationship between incest experienced during childhood and dysfunction in adult life. Of the total sample, almost 30% of the women had experienced incest, and of that group, 40% met the criteria for PTSD. In addition, these women were rated as significantly more depressed and exhibited a greater degree of anxiety than the nonincestuously abused women.

More recently, Donaldson and Gardner (1985) collected data from 26 women seen clinically who had experienced incest as children. Presenting symptoms included lack of sexual response, depressed feelings, anxiety attacks, and relationship difficulties. The *DSM-III* (American Psychiatric Association, 1980) diagnostic criteria for PTSD were used in evaluating the subject's case histories and symptom profiles. Results indicated that 25 of the 26 women met the diagnostic criteria for delayed or chronic PTSD (subtypes included in *DSM-III* criteria). In the third study, Lindberg and Distad (1985) treated 17 women who entered individual therapy with a variety of presenting complaints (none incest related). During the course of therapy, the history of abuse was disclosed. It was observed that the symptoms exhibited in this clinical population of women fit the features of a chronic or delayed post-traumatic stress disorder.

From these reports, it appears that some adult victims of childhood sexual abuse meet the criteria for a post-traumatic stress disorder. In Table 5.3, we have identified the PTSD symptoms that have been reported among adults abused as children (long-term effects). Regarding criterion A, many victims view their abusive experiences as being the most psychologically damaging of their lives (e.g., Lindberg & Distad, 1985). Incest has been compared, on a theoretical level, to the interminable existence of life in the concentration camps during World War II (Silver et al., 1983). The literature is also replete with evidence that abuse victims re-experience the trauma (criterion B). In addition, their symptoms are often exacerbated when they are exposed to events that resemble the original traumatic event, most notably participation in sexual activities. Almost all clinical studies document problems in victims related to sexual adjustment (Browne & Finkelhor, 1986).

Regarding criterion C, impaired emotionality is one of the most commonly reported symptoms among adults abused as children. Among others, depressive symptoms, suicidal ideation, and an inability to become emotionally close to other people in adulthood have all been reported by victims. It would appear that having had their basic trust violated during childhood, victims are unable to become close to or trust others later in life. Fearing the power of their emotions to destroy themselves and the offender, child victims instead mask their anger, sadness, and ambivalence toward the person who betrayed them. This resultant numbing leaves them detached from their own feelings. Detachment serves as a survival technique, to allow them to be in control.

Persistent avoidance of stimuli associated with trauma, an additional component of criterion C, is another symptom frequently reported among adults abused as children. Perhaps the most troublesome activity these victims avoid is becoming emotionally close to other people. Becoming close elicits uncomfortable feelings and many victims report having difficulty establishing intimate human relationships (Steele & Alexander, 1981; Tsai & Wagner, 1978). Other avoidant behaviors include evasion of men, psychogenic amnesia, and the use of dissociation as a psychological defense.

As adults, episodes of numbing have been conceptualized as the result of control efforts aimed at preventing intrusive ideas and feelings (Horowitz et al., 1980). When repetitive thoughts occur despite controls, the episodes will be experienced as intrusive. In contrast, when controls dominate and triggers to repetition are avoided, the result will be episodes of unusual constriction of ideational ranges, with dampening of emotional responsivity. The

DSM-III-R, like its predecessor, assumes that symptoms of intrusion, re-experiencing, numbing, and avoidance occur together. Recent work on PTSD among Vietnam veterans has developed some evidence that there is systematic variation in the types of stress symptoms in this population (Laufer, Brett, & Gallops, 1985). In contrast to the comprehensive model proposed in the *DSM-III-R*, a second model proposed by Laufer and associates (1985) hypothesizes that there are two distinct dimensions to the disorder: one concerning repetitions of ideational, affective, or somatic aspects of the trauma (re-experiencing); and the second related to efforts to avoid or defend against such repetitions (denial). It may be that different types of abuse-related experiences result in different patterns of stress symptoms as has been found regarding types of combat experiences. Alternatively, it may be that cross-sectional designs have obscured a developmental pattern of moving from denial to re-experiencing as suggested by the survivor theory (Horowitz & Solomon, 1975; Lifton, 1973). According to this theory, people exposed to severe trauma go through a latency or denial-numbing phase lasting from a few days to decades. This phase is followed by the intrusive-repetitive phase, where the victim begins to experience nightmares, frustration, and guilt. Adherence to the *DSM-III-R* requirement that re-experiencing and numbing symptoms occur simultaneously could hinder the identification of abuse victims and underestimate the prevalence of PTSD among them.

Strong support for the existence of symptoms listed in criterion D can be found. Victims frequently report being hyperalert and having difficulty sleeping and concentrating (e.g., Briere, 1984; Courtois & Watts, 1982; Lindberg & Distad, 1985). In addition, some adults abused as children display specific physiological reactions such as anxiety attacks (e.g., Briere, 1984). Finally, many victims exhibit symptoms listed in the "*Associated Features*" section, including suicidal ideation, symptoms of depression and anxiety, impulsive behaviors, headaches, and stomach problems. Feelings of guilt about their participation in the activity are also commonly reported.

In conclusion, it is apparent that PTSD is a pervasive disorder in victims of sexual abuse. Evidence is accumulating to indicate that the trauma associated with sexual abuse may manifest itself as PTSD in children and adolescents, and also in adults who were abused as children. That abuse victims have not been diagnosed in the past as having PTSD may be due to the fact that PTSD may be difficult to recognize and assess, perhaps because of the victim's young age, the range and severity of symptoms, or the victim's tendency to conceal both symptoms and the details of the abuse (Goodwin, 1985). Identification of PTSD in victims of sexual abuse has important implications for clinicians and researchers. In the following section, we will discuss the implications of sexual-abuse-related PTSD as they relate to clinical practice and research efforts in the area of childhood sexual abuse.

IMPLICATIONS

Conceptualizing the initial and long-term effects of sexual abuse as a post-traumatic stress disorder has several important implications for professionals who work with adults and children in general, those involved with victims of sexual abuse, and those conducting research in the area of sexual abuse. In this section, specific suggestions will be offered to aid clinicians in assessing and diagnosing adult and child victims of sexual abuse, to aid therapists in providing treatment interventions for sexually abused children and adults abused as children, and to aid researchers investigating sexual abuse and its traumatogenic effects.

ASSESSMENT

Perhaps part of the reason that sexual-abuse-related PTSD has been overlooked by clinicians working with child victims of sexual abuse is that child psychic trauma in general has been a neglected topic in the research literature. In evaluating this population, clinicians must first be willing to accept the existence of psychological sequelae in the child victim of trauma. Although the recently revised edition of the *DSM-III* addresses particular age-specific features of PTSD, no special diagnostic criteria applicable to traumatized children have been incorporated into the revision. Another impediment to diagnosis is the fact that the symptoms of sexual-abuse-related PTSD can be easily overlooked if clinicians fail to ask about child sexual abuse (Goodwin, 1985). We encourage clinicians to view the constellation of such symptoms in young children as depression, somatization, anxiety, sexualized behavior, or poor social functioning as the primary symptom complex associated with sexual-abuse-related PTSD. Young children should be asked in a sensitive and age-appropriate manner about sexual abuse whenever the above symptom complex is presented (Adams-Tucker, 1982). Direct questioning regarding sexually abusive experiences should be initiated with older children who present with such symptoms as withdrawal, poor social functioning, delinquency, runaway behavior, or substance abuse, which compose the primary symptom complex associated with PTSD in this group. Clinicians should also be aware that some sexually abused children may show none of the previous symptoms. Often there is a significant delay before the onset of PTSD symptoms (Terr, 1981b, 1983). For this reason, we recommend that all children be asked about exploitive sexual experiences during routine information gathering.

Perhaps another part of the problem in diagnosing PTSD in children relates to the fact that the development of child-oriented assessment protocols has lagged behind the work being conducted with adults (e.g., Blanchard et al., 1986; Malloy, Fairbank, & Keane, 1983; J. Wolfe et al., 1987). Unfortunately, very little empirical data exist on methods for systematically assessing PTSD in child abuse victims. Recently, V. V. Wolfe and D. A. Wolfe (1988) have provided guidelines and procedures for the behavioral assessment of the child sexual abuse victim and several of the recommended assessment methods would be appropriate for distinguishing PTSD victims from victims who do not have PTSD. For example, the Children's Impact of Traumatic Events Scale (V. V. Wolfe, D. A. Wolfe, & Larose, 1986) provides a structured format for interviewing children about their perceptions of the impact of the abuse and their attributions toward the abuse. It contains items related to intrusive thoughts and the child's perceptions of blame, guilt, betrayal, stigmatization, and helplessness. Early diagnosis of and intervention with sexual-abuse-related PTSD is imperative so that immediate distress is reduced, delayed responses may be prevented, and pathological responses may be abated before becoming fixed, making for a briefer intervention (Adams-Tucker, 1982; Caplan, 1964; Horowitz, 1986; Lindemann, 1944).

In evaluating adults, clinicians must be open to the possibility that emotional problems in some adults may be a long-term stress reaction to untreated sexual abuse trauma. Adults may show signs of other disorders or conceal early sexually abusive experiences. We encourage the inclusion of questions about such experiences during routine history taking with all adults. Such questioning affords the client an opportunity to disclose the abuse, as through the initiation of this sensitive topic, the therapist "normalizes" what may be in the client's mind a "taboo" topic. In addition, even if disclosure does not immediately follow with those clients who have been abused, asking may allow for later disclosure during the course of therapy (Alter-Reid et al., 1986).

Again, we encourage clinicians to view the constellation of such symptoms in adults as anxiety, depression, flashbacks, self-destructive behavior, eating disorders, or sexual interpersonal dysfunction as the primary symptom complex associated with sexual-abuse-related PTSD. Viewing the PTSD symptoms in isolation would most likely result in inappropriate diagnoses (e.g., generalized anxiety disorder, major depressive episode, dissociative disorder, borderline personality disorder) and delay the provision of appropriate treatment.

Similar to the state of affairs in child assessment of sexual-abuse-related PTSD, progress in the assessment of adults abused as children has been limited. There are several interview schedules available for assessing combat-related PTSD (e.g., Brecksville PTSD Inventory - Smith, 1985; Jackson Structured Interview - Keane et al., 1985), but there are no published structured interviews available for assessing civilian-related PTSD, with one exception - the PTSD subsection of the Structured Clinical Interview for *DSM-III* (SCID - Spitzer & Williams, 1985). However, as J. Wolfe and her colleagues (1987) point out, "the SCID subsection lacks careful documentation of pre- and post-trauma development and focuses primarily on obtaining sufficient current symptom information to determine whether an individual meets current DSM-III criteria for the PTSD diagnosis" (p. 30).

Recently, J. Wolfe et al. (1987) reviewed the PTSD assessment literature and recommended that a multimethod approach be employed that would include structured clinical interviews, psychometric tests, and psychophysiological evaluations. As part of their structured clinical interview, this group has found the Jackson Structured Interview (Keane et al., 1985) to be helpful and suggests its utility in evaluating adults sexually abused as children. The interview comprehensively reviews: (a) the current functioning of the individual, including background demographics, and educational, vocational, and social situations; (b) the factors related to the initiation of treatment, including important antecedent events and their consequences; and (c) the formation of symptom complexes (e.g., symptom severity, frequency, duration, and precipitating factors), along with the presence of clinical features specific to the symptoms of PTSD (e.g., anxiety, depression, re-experiencing the trauma, numbness, emotional withdrawal, and exaggerated startle response). In addition, J. Wolfe et al. (1987) recommended that a careful mental status examination be given along with psychometric testing (e.g., MMPI - Hathaway & McKinley, 1967; STAI - Spielberger, Gorsuch, & Lushene, 1970).

Recently, several authors have suggested the inclusion of a psychophysiological evaluation component in assessing PTSD (Davidson & Baum, 1986; J. Wolfe et al., 1987). In general, this component includes varied measures of physiological arousal (e.g., heart rate) on responses to stimuli (e.g., unexpected loud noise or sudden physical contact) believed to be associated with the phobic or startle reaction symptom of PTSD. The inclusion of this assessment procedure is consistent with recent formulations of PTSD as representing an extreme form of the human organism's integrated psychophysiological response to stress involving sympathetic arousal (Davidson & Baum, 1986).

Thus, an essential first step in assisting victims with this debilitating syndrome is to conduct a careful, comprehensive assessment. A thorough evaluation provides a basis for the clinical determination of the presence and scope of PTSD, which subsequently leads to the development of an appropriate therapeutic intervention. Multimethod assessment approaches are recommended and further development and refinement of assessment methods are needed. Assessment procedures might include information obtained from structured interviews, self-report measures, psychometric instruments, projective techniques, behavioral and psychophysiological measures, and reports of family members and friends where indicated. A multimethod assessment approach is advantageous as it provides information from a wide variety of sources, allows for inspection of the convergence of information (J. Wolfe et al., 1987), and provides detailed information helpful in delineating the many and often diverse components of sexual-abuse-related PTSD.

More specifically, the clinician's evaluation must appraise not only the degree of external stress imposed (e.g., duration and frequency of abuse, type of sexual act encountered, etc.), but also the degree of stress experienced by the victim (e.g., the affective nature of the relationship between perpetrator and victim, the victim's perceived responsibility, adverse reactions to disclosure experienced by the victim, etc.). In addition, the clinician should investigate the client's previctimization experiences, including his or her relationships with family, peers, and authority figures, and evaluate how the client's current stress experience interacts with the person's preexisting personality characteristics. In some instances, the existence of preabuse difficulties would suggest that a personality diagnosis would be the primary diagnosis. However, Eth and Pynoos (1985) have advised therapists to refrain from diagnosing personality disorders until posttraumatic symptoms have abated. Finally, along with premorbid variables and current stress experiences, the clinician should consider the social and environmental supports available to the client as well as his or her coping resources. Evaluating the interaction between the current stress experience and the client's coping resources is essential in determining treatment approaches and in estimating prognosis.

THERAPEUTIC INTERVENTION

Therapeutic goals for the sexual abuse victim suffering from PTSD should be similar to those set for Vietnam veterans suffering from PTSD (e.g., Horowitz, 1986; Williams, 1980). For example, victims should be encouraged to express their feelings about the abusive experience (Donaldson & Gardner, 1985; Giaretto, 1976; Lindberg & Distad, 1985). In order for this to occur, clinicians must begin treatment by establishing a safe and communicative relationship. However, therapists need to be aware that although client-therapist trust is important, it is difficult to develop because these victims have been deprived of basic trust during critical developmental phases.

For many children suffering from sexual-abuse-related PTSD, feelings about the experience are expressed indirectly through post-traumatic play or artwork that serves to defend the child from recalling intolerable emotions and memories (Jones, 1986; Terr, 1981b). As therapy progresses, the clinician may identify the type of feelings that seem to precipitate such play and reflect this to the child. The aim is to help the child become more aware of his or her emotional feelings and allow them to be ventilated (Jones, 1986).

For adult sufferers of sexual-abuse-related PTSD, providing them with the opportunity to express feelings related to the abuse experience helps to break the cyclical alternation of denial and intrusion by providing a safe environment in which they can experience the emotional response of the traumatic event(s) without automatic denial and numbing of the emotions (Horowitz, 1976). To overcome chronic feelings of numbness and isolation, clients need to tolerate and share the feelings associated with their memories of the abusive experience (Donaldson & Gardner, 1985). They need to be aware that as they break through the powerful denial, they are likely to experience intrusive-repetitious thoughts. The memories, perceptions about the memories, and feeling reactions must be experienced in tolerable doses. Victims may become anxious that these frightening experiences are occurring and may interpret them as a sign of losing control or "going crazy." Anticipating these reactions and providing support and reassurance when they do occur would be necessary. It is also important for the therapist to allow clients to maintain a balance between their denial and emotional reactions. Patients should be encouraged to retain as much voluntary control of the process as possible. As a result, the breakthrough of previously repressed material is experienced as active mastery rather than as repeated victimization (Herman & Schatzow, 1987).

Another goal of treatment is to help the client realize and accept that the abuse was the adult perpetrator's responsibility (Forward & Buck, 1978; Lindberg & Distad, 1985; Meiselman, 1978). An important component of this goal is the clinician's supportive reaction to the victim's disclosure. For many child and adult sexual abuse survivors, therapy will be the first opportunity for supported disclosure. For both children and adults, the clinician's first response must be to believe what the client is saying and to avoid an anxious overreaction that would confirm the client's belief that something is wrong with himself or herself (Swanson & Biaggio, 1985). Supportive disclosure can reduce negative self-evaluation, increase trust in others, and result in the client's eventually incorporating the trauma in a more adaptive manner as a function of

121

being given the opportunity to express feelings of self-blame, guilt, anger, and isolation with a safe and trusted person (Alter-Reid et al., 1986).

Therapeutic interventions with children aimed at relieving any guilt or sense of responsibility may include discussion of possible ambivalent feelings toward the offender or feelings of responsibility for changes in the family situation resulting from the child's disclosure of the abuse (Conte & Berliner, 1981). Child sexual abuse victims often experience guilt because they participated in or perceived some or all aspects of the experience as pleasurable. To help alleviate this guilt, the therapist may need to give the client "permission" to experience feelings of sexual pleasure or memories of participation (Jones, 1986). Explaining the pleasurable experiences as the body's normal reaction to sexual stimulation may also be helpful.

For the adult client experiencing guilt reactions, group therapy with other sexual abuse victims can be especially beneficial once the victim is able to think about the incest without being overwhelmed (Tsai & Wagner, 1978). Victimized group members may provide helpful reassurance that others have been victimized, that their participation in the abuse experience was not their fault, and that they were not responsible for the abuse. In addition, as the victims become able to recall the event and experience less intense emotional reactions, the therapeutic focus can switch to helping them modify their misconceptions about the event (e.g., the person's attributions regarding the abuse; switching from "I am responsible for the incest - I caused it" to "I am not responsible for the incest - I was a victim"). Recent applications of the learned helplessness phenomenon to explain the emotional numbing, maladaptive helplessness and passivity, and loss of self-esteem seen in many abuse-related PTSD victims can also provide clinicians with a framework in which to focus on changing victims' attributions regarding the abuse (Gold, 1986; Peterson & Seligman, 1983). Cognitive therapy techniques could be used to explore attributional style, modify self-defeating thoughts, and help victims develop a sense of mastery and control over their lives.

Two additional goals of therapy are to aid the client in (a) understanding how the abuse led to current self-defeating behavioral patterns, and (b) learning new adaptive behaviors (Lindberg & Distad, 1985). The therapist's role is to explore with the client each symptom component of the PTSD, emphasizing the damaging role that the sexually abusive experience played in symptom development. As Herman and Schatzow (1987) point out, the purpose of reliving the experience is not simply one of catharsis, but also of integration. By exploring self-defeating behavioral patterns and symptomatology, previously confusing symptomatology, feelings, and behaviors become understandable to the client and he or she is thus able to integrate and comprehend past abusive experiences and their impact on present life circumstances. In addition, as the client comes to understand how the sexual abuse trauma contributed to his or her symptoms (e.g., withdrawal, social dysfunction, antisocial, or acting-out behaviors, sexual maladjustment, depression, poor self-esteem, etc.), the client can then learn new behaviors and slowly change self-defeating behavioral patterns (Lindberg & Distad, 1985). As he or she learns new adaptive behaviors, stress is reduced and self-esteem is increased as the client is given a new sense of power and control over his or her life.

In conclusion, therapists working with children and adults suffering from sexual-abuse-related PTSD need to afford these victims a safe environment in which to express feelings, and to provide them with a way to conceptualize thoughts, behaviors, and feelings, and to enhance their sense of power, control, and hope.

RESEARCH ISSUES

We have identified some important guidelines and procedures that should prove helpful in the assessment, diagnosis, and treatment of sexual-abuse-related PTSD in adults and children. However, more empirical research is needed in this area to refine current approaches, to develop new multimethod assessments, and to determine which treatment approaches are most appropriate and effective. Additional research is required to determine the validity of the sexual-abuse-related PTSD diagnosis, differences between the child and adult presentations of the disorder, how the stress symptom features are exacerbated if the syndrome is not dealt with immediately (Donaldson & Gardner, 1985), and qualitative differences among sexual-abuse-related PTSD, combat-related PTSD, and other civilian-related PTSDs. Treatment outcome research using standardized measures is greatly needed. In addition, follow-up evaluations to assure the stability of treatment effects should be conducted.

Clearly, not all sexually abused children experience PTSD, nor do all adults abused as children. Future research should investigate risk factors associated with the development of sexual-abuse-related PTSD. In the child sexual abuse literature, several initial investigations suggest a relationship between characteristics of the sexual abuse experience (e.g., duration and frequency of abuse, type of sexual act encountered, affective nature of the relationship between perpetrator and victim, etc.) and the psychological effect on the victim (e.g., Conte & Schuerman, 1987; Herman, Russell, & Trocki, 1986). Perhaps elements of the abusive experience interact with other factors (e.g., the individual's coping resources, victim perception of the event, previctimization adjustment) to determine the kind and degree of PTSD that results. Research on combat-related PTSD suggests that the amount and intensity of combat and other variables (e.g., social support systems, unemployment, instability of family origin, etc.) interact to produce varying degrees of PTSD (Foy et al., 1984; Norman, 1982). In a similar vein, researchers need to determine the particular characteristics of the sexual trauma and other variables (e.g., developmental stage of victim, defense mechanisms employed, etc.) necessary to cause PTSD. Finally, researchers and clinicians need to determine which of these factors can be prevented, or at least altered, by specific treatment approaches. Such efforts should help to decrease the suffering experienced by sexual abuse victims and should contribute to our understanding of childhood sexual abuse and its traumatogenic effects.

Cindy L. Miller-Perrin, MS, earned her BA degree in psychology at Pepperdine University, Malibu, California in 1983. In 1984 she began her doctoral studies at Washington State University, Pullman, earning her MS degree in clinical psychology in 1987. She recently completed her dissertation which focused on cognitive mediators affecting the psychological impact of sexual abuse and will receive her PhD from Washington State University in 1991, following her clinical internship. Ms. Miller-Perrin may be contacted at the Psychology Department, Johnson Tower, Washington State University, Pullman, WA 99164.

Sandy K. Wurtele, PhD, earned her doctorate at The University of Alabama in clinical child psychology. Following her clinical internship at the University of Mississippi Medical Center in Jackson, she taught for 5 years at Washington State University. Dr. Wurtele is now at the University of Colorado where she holds a FIRST Award from the National Institute of Mental Health to conduct research on child sexual abuse and its prevention. Dr. Wurtele can be contacted at the Psychology Department, University of Colorado, Colorado Springs, CO 80933-7150.

REFERENCES

Achenbach, T. M., & Edelbrock, C. (1983). *Manual for the Child Behavior Checklist.* Burlington: University of Vermont.

Adams-Tucker, C. (1981). A socioclinical overview of 28 sex-abused children. *Child Abuse & Neglect, 5,* 361-367.

Adams-Tucker, C. (1982). Proximate effects of sexual abuse in childhood: A report on 28 children. *American Journal of Psychiatry, 139,* 1252-1256.

Adams-Tucker, C. (1985). Defense mechanisms used by sexually abused children. *Children Today, 34,* 9-12.

Alter-Reid, K., Gibbs, M. S., Lachenmeyer, J. R., Sigal, J., & Massoth, N. A. (1986). Sexual abuse of children: A review of the empirical findings. *Clinical Psychology Review, 6,* 249-266.

American Psychiatric Association. (1980). *Diagnostic and Statistical Manual of Mental Disorders* (3rd ed.). Washington, DC: Author.

American Psychiatric Association. (1987). *Diagnostic and Statistical Manual of Mental Disorders* (3rd ed. rev.). Washington, DC: Author.

Anderson, S. C., Bach, C. M., & Griffith, S. (1981, April). *Psychosocial Sequelae in Intrafamilial Victims of Sexual Assault and Abuse.* Paper presented at the Third International Conference on Child Abuse and Neglect, Amsterdam, The Netherlands.

Bagley, C., & Ramsay, R. (1985, February). *Disrupted Childhood and Vulnerability to Sexual Assault: Long-Term Sequels with Implications for Counseling.* Paper presented at the Conference on Counseling the Sexual Abuse Survivor, Winnipeg, Canada.

Bender, L., & Blau, A. (1937). The reaction of children to sexual relationships with adults. *American Journal of Orthopsychiatry, 7,* 500-518.

Bender, L., & Grugett, A. E. (1952). Incest: A synthesis of data. *American Journal of Orthopsychiatry, 12,* 825-837.

Benedek, E. D. (1985). Children and disaster: Emerging issues. *Psychiatric Annals, 15,* 168-172.

Blanchard, E. B., Gerardi, R. J., Kolb, L. C., & Barlow, D. H. (1986). The utility of the anxiety disorders interview schedule (ADIS) in the diagnosis of post-traumatic stress disorder (PTSD) in Vietnam veterans. *Behavioral Research, 24,* 577-580.

Branch, G., & Paxton, R. (1965). A study of gynococcal infections among infants and children. *Public Health Reports, 80,* 347.

Brandt, R., & Tisza, V. (1977). The sexually misused child. *American Journal of Orthopsychiatry, 47,* 80-90.

Briere, J. (1984, April). *The Effects of Childhood Sexual Abuse on Later Psychological Functioning: Defining a "Post-Sexual-Abuse Syndrome."* Paper presented at the Third National Conference on Sexual Victimization of Children, Washington, DC.

Briere, J., & Runtz, M. (1985, August). *Symptomatology Associated with Prior Sexual Abuse in a Nonclinical Sample.* Paper presented at the annual meeting of the American Psychological Association, Los Angeles, CA.

Briere, J., & Runtz, M. (1986). Suicidal thoughts and behaviors in former sexual abuse victims. *Canadian Journal of Behavioral Sciences, 18,* 413-423.

Browne, A., & Finkelhor, D. (1986). Impact of child sexual abuse: A review of the research. *Psychological Bulletin, 99,* 66-77.

Browning, D. H., & Boatman, B. (1977). Incest: Children at risk. *American Journal of Psychiatry, 134,* 69-72.

Burgess, A. W., Groth, A. N., & McCausland, M. (1981). Child sex initiation rings. *American Journal of Orthopsychiatry, 51,* 110-119.

Burgess, A. W., Hartman, C. R., McCausland, M. P., & Powers, P. (1984). Response patterns in children and adolescents exploited through sex rings and pornography. *American Journal of Psychiatry, 141,* 656-662.

Burgess, A. W., & Holmstrom, L. L. (1975). Sexual trauma of children and adolescents: Pressure, sex, and secrecy. *Nursing Clinics of North America, 10,* 551-563.

Burton, L. (1968). *Vulnerable Children.* London: Routledge & Kegal Paul.

Caplan, G. (1964). *Principles of Preventive Psychiatry.* New York: Basic Books.

Conte, J. R., & Berliner, L. (1981). Sexual abuse of children: Implications for practice. *Social Casework: The Journal of Contemporary Social Work, 62,* 601-606.

Conte, J. R., & Schuerman, J. R. (1987). Factors associated with an increased impact of child sexual abuse. *Child Abuse & Neglect, 11,* 201-211.

Courtois, C. A. (1979, Nov.-Dec.). Characteristics of a volunteer sample of adult women who experienced incest in childhood and adolescence. *Dissertation Abstracts International, 40A,* 3194-A.

Courtois, C. A. (1980). Studying and counseling women with past incest experience. *Victimology: An International Journal, 5,* 322-334.

Courtois, C. A., & Watts, D. L. (1982). Counseling adult women who had experienced incest in childhood or adolescence. *Personnel and Guidance Journal, 60,* 275-279.

Davidson, L. M., & Baum, A. (1986). Chronic stress and posttraumatic stress disorders. *Journal of Consulting and Clinical Psychology, 54,* 303-308.

DeFrancis, V. (1969). *Protecting the Child Victim of Sex Crimes Committed by Adults.* Denver, CO: American Humane Association.

de Young, M. (1982). Innocent seducer or innocently seduced? The role of the child incest victim. *Journal of Clinical Child Psychology, 11,* 56-60.

Dixon, K. N., Arnold, L. E., & Calestro, K. (1978). Father-son incest: Underreported psychiatric problem. *American Journal of Psychiatry, 135,* 835-838.

Donaldson, M. A., & Gardner, R. (1985). Diagnosis and treatment of traumatic stress among women after childhood incest. In C. Figley (Ed.), *Trauma and Its Wake* (pp. 356-377). New York: Brunner/Mazel.

Eth, S., & Pynoos, R. S. (1985). *Post-Traumatic Stress Disorder in Children.* Washington, DC: American Psychiatric Press.

Everstine, D. S., & Everstine, L. (Eds.). (1983). *People in Crisis: Strategic Therapeutic Interventions.* New York: Brunner/Mazel.

Fagan, J., & McMahon, P. P. (1984). Incipient multiple personality in children: Four cases. *Journal of Nervous Mental Disorders, 172,* 26-36.

Ferenczi, S. (1949). Confusion of tongues between adult and child. *International Journal of Psychoanalysis, 30,* 225.

Finkelhor, D. (1979). *Sexually Victimized Children.* New York: Free Press.

Forbes, L. M. (1972). Incest, anger, and suicide. In I. H. Berkovitz (Ed.), *Adolescents Grow in Groups: Clinical Experiences in Adolescent Group Psychotherapy* (pp. 104-107). New York: Brunner/Mazel.

Forward, S., & Buck, C. (1978). *Betrayal of Innocence: Incest and Its Devastation.* Los Angeles: J. P. Tarcher.

Foy, D. W., Sipprelle, R. C., Rueger, D. B., & Carroll, E. M. (1984). Etiology of PTSD in Vietnam veterans: An analysis of preliminary, military, and combat exposure influences. *Journal of Consulting and Clinical Psychology, 52,* 79-81.

Friedrich, W. N., Urquiza, A. J., & Beilke, R. (1986). Behavioral problems in sexually abused young children. *Journal of Pediatric Psychology, 11,* 47-57.

Fromuth, M. E. (1986). The relationship of childhood sexual abuse with later psychological adjustment in a sample of college women. *Child Abuse & Neglect, 10,* 5-15.

Gagnon, J. (1965). Female child victims of sex offenses. *Social Problems, 13,* 176-192.

Gelinas, D. J. (1983). The persisting negative effects of incest. *Psychiatry, 46,* 312-332.

Giaretto, H. (1976). Humanistic treatment of father-daughter incest. In R. Helfer & H. Kempe (Eds.), *Child Abuse and Neglect: The Family and the Community* (pp. 143-162). Cambridge, MA: Ballinger Publishing Co.

Gislason, I. L., & Call, J. D. (1982). Dog bite in infancy: Trauma and personality development. *Journal of American Academy of Child Psychiatry, 21,* 203-207.

Gold, E. R. (1986). Long-term effects of sexual victimization in childhood: An attributional approach. *Journal of Consulting and Clinical Psychology, 54,* 471-475.

Gomes-Schwartz, B., Horowitz, M. J., & Sauzier, M. (1985). Severity of emotional distress among sexually abused preschool, school-age, and adolescent children. *Hospital and Community Psychiatry, 36,* 503-508.

Goodwin, J. (1985). Post-traumatic symptoms in incest victims. In R. Pynoos & S. Eth (Eds.). *Post-Traumatic Stress Disorder in Children* (pp. 157-168). Washington, DC: American Psychiatric Press.

Goodwin, J., McCarthy, T., & DiVasto, P. (1981). Prior incest in mothers of abused children. *Child Abuse & Neglect, 5,* 87-96.

Guyon, R. (1941). *Ethics of Sexual Acts.* New York: Blue Ribbon.

Harrison, P. A., Lumry, A. E., & Claypatch, C. (1984, August). *Female Sexual Abuse Victims: Perspectives on Family Dysfunction, Substance Use and Psychiatric Disorders.* Paper presented at the Second National Conference for Family Violence Researchers, Durham, NH.

Hathaway, S. E., & McKinley, T. C. (1967). *Minnesota Multiphasic Personality Inventory: Manual for Administration and Scoring.* New York: Psychological Corporation.

Henderson, D. J. (1972). Incest: A synthesis of data. *Canadian Psychiatric Association Journal, 17,* 299-313.

Henderson, J. (1983). Is incest harmful? *Canadian Journal of Psychiatry, 28,* 34-40.

Herman, J. L. (1981). *Father-Daughter Incest.* Cambridge, MA: Harvard University Press.

Herman, J., & Hirschman, L. (1981). Families at risk for father-daughter incest. *American Journal of Psychiatry, 138,* 967-970.

Herman, J., Russell, D., & Trocki, K. (1986). Long-term effects of incestuous abuse in childhood. *American Journal of Psychiatry, 143,* 1293-1296.

Herman, J. L., & Schatzow, E. (1987). Recovery and verification of memories of childhood sexual trauma. *Psychoanalytic Psychology, 4,* 1-14.

Horowitz, M. J. (1976). *Stress-Response Syndromes.* New York: Jason Aronson.

Horowitz, M. J. (1986). Stress-response syndromes: A review of post-traumatic and adjustment disorders. *Hospital and Community Psychiatry, 37,* 241-249.

Horowitz, M. J., & Solomon, G. F. (1975). Prediction of delayed stress response syndrome in Vietnam veterans. *Journal of Social Issues, 31,* 67-80.

Horowitz, M. J., Wilner, M., Kaltreider, N., & Alvarez, W. (1980). Signs and symptoms of post-traumatic stress disorder. *Archives of General Psychiatry, 37,* 85-92.

Isaacs, S. (1933). *Social Development of Young Children.* London: Routledge.

James, J., & Meyerding, J. (1977). Early sexual experience as a factor in prostitution. *Archives of Sexual Behavior, 17,* 31-42.

Jones, D. P. H. (1986). Individual psychotherapy for the sexually abused child. *Child Abuse & Neglect, 10,* 377-385.

Justice, B., & Justice, R. (1979). *The Broken Taboo: Sex in the Family.* New York: Human Sciences Press.

Katan, A. (1973). Children who were raped. *The Psychoanalytic View of the Child, 28,* 208-224.

Kaufman, I., Peck, A., & Tagiuri, C. (1954). The family constellation and overt incestuous relations between father and daughter. *American Journal of Orthopsychiatry, 24,* 266-279.

Keane, T. M., Fairbank, J. A., Caddell, J. M., Zimering, R. T., & Bender, M. E. (1985). A behavioral approach to assessing and treating PTSD in Vietnam veterans. In C. R. Figley (Ed.), *Trauma and Its Wake* (pp. 257-294). New York: Brunner/Mazel.

Kinsey, A. C., Pomeroy, W. B., Martin, C. E., & Gebhard, P. H. (1953). *Sexual Behavior in the Human Female.* Philadelphia: Saunders.

Kluft, R. (1984). Treatment of multiple personality disorder: A study of 33 cases. *Psychiatric Clinics of North America, 7,* 9-30.

Kovach, J. (1983). The relationship between treatment failures of alcoholic women and incestuous histories with possible implications for post-traumatic stress disorder symptomatology. *Dissertation Abstracts International, 44,* 710-A.

Lacey, G. (1972). Observations on Aberfan. *Journal of Psychosomatic Research, 16,* 257-260.

Langmade, C. J. (1983). The impact of pre- and post-pubertal onset of incest experiences in adult women as measured by sex anxiety, sex guilt, sexual satisfaction and sexual behavior. *Dissertation Abstracts International, 44,* 917B. (University Microfilms No. 3592)

Laufer, R. S., Brett, E., & Gallops, M. S. (1985). Symptom patterns associated with posttraumatic stress disorder among Vietnam veterans exposed to war trauma. *American Journal of Psychiatry, 142,* 1304-1311.

Lewis, M., & Sarrell, P. M. (1969). Some psychological aspects of seduction, incest and rape in childhood. *Journal of the American Academy of Child Psychiatry, 8,* 606.

Lifton, R. J. (1973). *Home From the War.* New York: Simon & Schuster.

Lindberg, F. H., & Distad, L. J. (1985). Post-traumatic stress disorders in women who experienced childhood incest. *Child Abuse & Neglect, 9,* 329-334.

Lindemann, E. (1944). Symptomatology and management of acute grief. *American Journal of Psychiatry, 101,* 141-148.

Lukianowicz, N. (1972). Incest I: Paternal incest. *British Journal of Psychiatry, 120,* 301-313.

Lusk, R., & Waterman, J. (1986). Effects of sexual abuse on children. In K. MacFarlane & J. Waterman (Eds.), *Sexual Abuse of Young Children* (pp. 101-113). New York: Guilford.

MacFarlane, K. (1978). Sexual abuse of children. In J. R. Chapman & M. Gates (Eds.), *Victimization of Women* (pp. 81-109). Beverly Hills, CA: Sage Publications.

MacFarlane, K., & Waterman, J. (Eds.). (1986). *Sexual Abuse of Young Children.* New York: Guilford.

Maisch, H. (1972). *Incest.* New York: Stein and Day.

Malloy, P. F., Fairbank, J. A., & Keane, T. M. (1983). Validation of multi-method assessment of post-traumatic stress disorders in Vietnam veterans. *Journal of Consulting and Clinical Psychology, 51,* 488-494.

Mannarino, A. P., & Cohen, J. A. (1986). A clinical-demographic study of sexually abused children. *Child Abuse & Neglect, 10,* 17-23.

Masson, J. M. (1984). *The Assault on Truth: Freud's Suppression of the Seduction Theory.* New York: Farrar, Straus, & Giroux.

Mehta, M. N., Lokeshwar, M. R., Bhatt, S. C., Athavale, V. B., & Kalkarni, B. S. (1979). Rape in children. *Child Abuse & Neglect, 3,* 671.

Meiselman, K. C. (1978). *Incest: A Psychological Study of Causes and Effects with Treatment Recommendations.* San Francisco: Jossey-Bass.

Mian, M., Wehrspann, W., Klajner-Diamond, H., LeBaron, D., & Winder, C. (1986). Review of 125 children 6 years of age and under who were sexually abused. *Child Abuse & Neglect, 10,* 223-229.

Miller, L. C. (1981). *Louisville Behavior Checklist.* Los Angeles: Western Psychological Services.

Mrazek, P. B. (1983). Sexual abuse of children. In B. B. Lahey & A. E. Kazdin (Eds.), *Advances in Clinical Child Psychology* (Vol. 6, pp. 199-215). New York: Plenum.

Mrazek, P. B., & Mrazek, D. A. (1981). The effects of child sexual abuse: Methodological considerations. In P. B. Mrazek & C. H. Kempe (Eds.), *Sexually Abused Children and Their Families* (pp. 235-245). New York: Pergamon.

Nakashima, I. I., & Zakus, G. E. (1977). Incest: Review and clinical experience. *Pediatrics, 60,* 696-701.

Nakashima, I. I., & Zakus, G. (1979). Incestuous families. *Pediatric Annals, 8,* 300-308.

Newman, C. J. (1976). Children of disaster: Clinical observations at Buffalo Creek. *American Journal of Psychiatry, 133,* 306-312.

Nielson, T. (1983). Sexual abuse of boys: Current perspectives. *The Personnel and Guidance Journal, 62,* 139-142.

Norman, E. M. (1982). The victims. *American Journal of Nursing, 82,* 1696-1698.

Oppenheimer, R., Palmer, R. L., & Brandon, S. (1984, September). *A Clinical Evaluation of Early Abusive Experiences in Adult Anorexic and Bulimic Females: Implications for Preventive Work in Childhood.* Paper presented at the Fifth International Congress on Child Abuse and Neglect, Montreal, Canada.

Peters, J. J. (1974). The psychological effects of childhood rape. *World Journal of Psychosynthesis, 6,* 11.

Peters, J. J. (1976). Children who are victims of sexual assault--The psychology of offenders. *American Journal of Psychotherapy, 30,* 398-421.

Peters. S. D. (1984). *The Relationship Between Childhood Sexual Victimization and Adult Depression among Afro-American and White Women.* Unpublished doctoral dissertation, University of California, Los Angeles, CA.

Peterson, C., & Seligman, M. E. P. (1983). Learned helplessness and victimization. *Journal of Social Issues, 39,* 103-116.

Putnam, F. (1984). The psychophysiologic investigation of multiple personality disorder. *Psychiatric Clinics of North America, 7,* 31-40.

Rabinovitch, R. D. (1953). Etiological factors in disturbed sexual behavior in children. *Journal of Criminal Law and Criminology, 43,* 610-621.

Rhinehart, J. W. (1961). Genesis of overt incest. *Comprehensive Psychiatry, 2,* 338.

Riggs, R. S. (1982). Incest: The school's role. *Journal of Social Health, 52,* 365-370.

Rosenfeld, A. A., Nadelson, C. C., & Krieger, M. (1979). Fantasy and reality in patients' reports of incest. *Journal of Clinical Psychiatry, 40,* 159-164.

Russell, D. E. H. (1986). *The Secret Trauma: Incest in the Lives of Girls and Women.* New York: Basic Books.

Sachs, R., Goodwin, J., & Braun, B. (in press). The role of childhood abuse in the development of multiple personality disorder. In B. Braun & R. Kluft (Eds.),

Multiple Personality and Dissociation. New York: Guilford.

Sedney, M. A., & Brooks, B. (1984). Factors associated with a history of childhood sexual experience in a nonclinical female population. *Journal of the American Academy of Child Psychiatry, 23,* 215-218.

Senior, N., Gladstone, T., & Nurcombe, B. (1982). Child snatching: A case report. *Journal of American Academy of Child Psychiatry, 20,* 579-583.

Shaw, V. L., & Meier, J. H. (1983). *The Effect of Type of Abuse and Neglect on Children's Psychosocial Development.* Unpublished manuscript, Children's Village U.S.A.

Silbert, M. H., & Pines, A. M. (1981). Sexual child abuse as an antecedent to prostitution. *Child Abuse & Neglect, 5,* 407-411.

Silver, R. L., Boon, C., & Stones, S. M. H. (1983). Searching for meaning in misfortune: Making sense of incest. *Journal of Social Issues, 39,* 81-102.

Sloane, P., & Karpinski, E. (1942). Effects of incest on the participants. *American Journal of Orthopsychiatry, 12,* 666-673.

Smith, J. (1985). *Brecksville Psychological Assessment Manual.* Unpublished manuscript.

Spielberger, C. D., Gorsuch, R. L., & Lushene, R. E. (1970). *Manual for the State-Trait Anxiety Inventory (Self-Evaluation Questionnaire).* Palo Alto, CA: Consultant Psychologists Press.

Spitzer, R. L., & Williams, J. B. (1985). *Structured Clinical Interview for DSM-III-R, Patient Version.* New York: Biometrics Research Department, New York State Psychiatric Institute.

Steele, B. F., & Alexander, H. (1981). Long-term effects of sexual abuse in childhood. In P. B. Mrazek & C. H. Kempe (Eds.), *Sexually Abused Children and Their Families* (pp. 223-234). New York: Pergamon.

Summit, R. C. (1983). The child sexual abuse accommodation syndrome. *Child Abuse & Neglect, 7,* 177-193.

Swanson, L., & Biaggio, M. K. (1985). Therapeutic perspectives on father-daughter incest. *American Journal of Psychiatry, 142,* 667-674.

Terr, L. C. (1979). Children of Chowchilla: A study of psychic trauma. *Psychoanalytic Study of Children, 34,* 547-623.

Terr, L. C. (1981a). Psychic trauma in children: Observations following the Chowchilla schoolbus kidnapping. *American Journal of Psychiatry, 138*, 14-19.

Terr, L. C. (1981b). Forbidden games: Post-traumatic child's play. *Journal of the American Academy of Child Psychiatry, 20*, 741-760.

Terr, L. C. (1983). Chowchilla revisited: The effects of psychic trauma four years after a school-bus kidnapping. *American Journal of Psychiatry, 140*, 1543-1550.

Terr, L. C. (1985). Psychic trauma in children and adolescents. *Psychiatric Clinics of North America, 8*, 815-835.

Tilelli, J. A., Tarek, D., & Jaffe, A. C. (1980). Sexual abuse of children: Clinical findings and implications for management. *New England Journal of Medicine, 302*, 319-323.

Tsai, M., Feldman-Summers, S., & Edgar, M. (1979). Childhood molestation: Variables related to differential impact of psychosexual functioning in adult women. *Journal of Abnormal Psychology, 88*, 407-417.

Tsai, M., & Wagner, N. N. (1978). Therapy groups for women sexually molested as children. *Archives of Sexual Behavior, 7*, 417-427.

Tufts' New England Medical Center, Division of Child Psychiatry. (1984). *Sexually Exploited Children: Service and Research Project.* Final report for the Office of Juvenile Justice and Delinquency Prevention. Washington, DC: Department of Justice.

Van Buskirk, S. S., & Cole, C. F. (1983). Characteristics of eight women seeking therapy for the effects of incest. *Psychotherapy: Theory, Research, and Practice, 20*, 503-514.

Weiss, J., Rogers, E., Darwin, M. R., & Dutton, D. E. (1955). A study of girl sex victims. *Psychiatric Quarterly, 29*, 1-26.

Williams, T. (1980). Therapeutic alliance and goal setting in the treatment of Vietnam veterans. In T. Williams (Ed.), *Post-Traumatic Stress Disorders of the Vietnam Veteran* (pp. 25-35). Cincinnati, OH: Disabled American Veterans.

Wolfe, J., Keane, T. M., Lyons, J. A., & Gerardi, R. J. (1987). Current trends and issues in the assessment of combat-related post-traumatic stress disorder. *The Behavior Therapist, 10*, 27-32.

Wolfe, V. V., & Wolfe, D. A. (1988). The sexually abused child. In E. J. Mash & L. G. Terdal (Eds.). *Behavioral*

Assessment of Childhood Disorders (2nd ed., pp. 670-714). New York: Guilford.

Wolfe, V. V., Wolfe, D. A., & Larose, L. (1986). *The Children's Impact of Traumatic Events Scale (CITES)*. Unpublished manuscript available from the authors at the Department of Psychology, the University of Western Ontario, London, Ontario, Canada N6A 5C2.

Yates, A. (1978). *Sex Without Shame: Encouraging the Child's Healthy Sexual Development.* New York: William Morrow & Co.

Yorukoglu, A., & Kemph, J. P. (1966). Children not severely damaged by incest with a parent. *Journal of the American Academy of Child Psychiatry, 5,* 111.

6.

Imagined, Exaggerated, and Malingered Post-Traumatic Stress Disorder

Emmett Early

Post-traumatic stress disorder (PTSD) is a difficult diagnosis to make with certainty. It is a diagnosis based largely on symptoms that are reported by the client rather than observed by the clinician (American Psychiatric Association, 1987; Resnick, 1984, p. 34). Although sleep disturbance is perhaps the only consistent, objectively measurable symptom (Hefez, Metz, & Lavie, 1987; Lavie et al., 1979; van der Kolk et al., 1984), it is not required for the diagnosis. The revised third edition of the *Diagnostic and Statistical Manual of Mental Disorders* (*DSM-III-R*) has added an item under category D, "Persistent symptoms of physiologic arousal": "physiologic reactivity upon exposure to events that symbolize or resemble an aspect of the traumatic event . . ." (American Psychiatric Association, 1987, p. 250). This symptom could also be regarded as objectively measurable, except that it is rarely a constant symptom, and really offers more potential as a research variable, as Kolb (1987) recently reviewed.

Because it is connected with big, unusual events that are often coupled with physical injuries, PTSD is the frequent subject of legal action, both criminal and civil, and an issue in claims for compensation and benefits (Erlinder, 1983; Raifman, 1983). Post-traumatic stress disorder, however, is also the result of an event that is outside the course of usual human experience. Thus, this disorder attracts people with identity confusion (Akhtar, 1984; Cohen, 1981; Diamond, 1971) and persons seeking a sympathetic patient role (Phillips, Ward, & Ries, 1983; Resnick, 1984; cf., Spiro, 1968, the history of trauma in Münchausen's syndrome). Yet, while it is attractive to those who are opportunistic or who would imagine themselves disordered, PTSD is also a sensitive diagnostic problem. Ordinary forensic methods that are often effective in identifying malingerers, such as repeated, rapid questioning, the identification of contradictions, and the presence of extreme or rare symptomatology (Rogers, 1986), become less useful when dealing with PTSD. An event that leads to trauma is often very confusing for the survivor to recall. Details may seem unreal (Horowitz, 1985). Indeed, clinicians have cautioned evaluators of trauma survivors to be alert for self-reporters who present confusing and often self-disclamatory details during the acute trauma phase, such as the rape survivor who discloses in her report that she should never have trusted the man, or the accident victim who criticizes his own judgment (Burgess & Holmstrom, 1979; Symonds, 1980; Titchener, 1970).

The recent publicity in the lay media regarding post-traumatic stress disorder and Vietnam veterans has led to national dissemination of PTSD criteria. Information about PTSD has been further promulgated by other victim advocacy groups (Atkinson, Henderson, & Sparr, 1982; Goodwin, undated; LaGuardia et al., 1983). Coupled with this notoriety is the confounding aspect of delayed PTSD with reports of symptoms appearing as late as 30 years after the traumatogenic event (Mayfield & Fowler, 1969; Solomon et al., 1987; Van Dyke, Zilberg, & McKinnon, 1985). Facts as basic as when and where an event occurred, particularly for cases that are remote in etiology, present forensic nightmares. For example, the traumas of wartime are many, frequently bizarre, and often poorly documented (Early, 1984; Scurfield & Blank, 1986). Confronting the patient regarding the reality of an alleged traumatogenic event may lead to the diagnosis of factitious PTSD (Sparr & Pankratz, 1983), or to further victimization of the survivor, as happened to many of the survivors of the nazi Holocaust (Krystal, 1967, p. 168) and others caught in prolonged proceedings for claims and compensation (Stern, 1976).

A hypothetical example of the effect of others' denial on the trauma survivor is a case in which a child is sexually molested by a parent, who, together with his spouse, denies the behavior. The child proceeds to repress the traumatic symptoms of fear and arousal and becomes a behavior problem. The original trauma events then become a pseudo-reality and the behavior problems are treated symptomatically. The symptoms of the trauma become chronic and the child begins using drugs. The sexual trauma continues to be denied (referred to as a "cop-out" by the drug counselors), and the trauma symptoms then become the source of mislabeled pathology.

A second example concerns a Vietnam veteran who survives an illegal mission into Cambodia, during which all of his friends are killed. The army denies such a mission took place. No one talks about it and nothing is noted in his military records. His anger at officers grows explosively, and he is given a bad conduct discharge for being absent without leave from a stateside assignment. He is denied his Veterans Administration (VA) benefits and the discharge appeals board refuses to listen to his trauma stories. His nightmares are so routine and concrete that he stops reporting them. The trauma has become a private event populated by characters and grizzly details that only exist in his mind.

In both examples, the reality of the traumatic event is denied by influential professionals. The behaviors that have developed secondary to the trauma are now, therefore, identified as symptoms of a personality disorder and treated as such. When the trauma is denied by professionals and others connected with the event, the survivor comes to doubt the reality and, albeit with anger, accepts the onus of having psychopathology of unknown etiology. Wilmer (1982) gives an excellent case study of this process resulting in a diagnosis of schizophrenia.

DIFFERENTIAL DIAGNOSIS

The first step in establishing PTSD as a diagnosis is the determination of the existence of a potentially traumatic event (i.e., a "recognizable stressor"). In a routine initial interview, trauma is surveyed by such questions as: "Have you had any near-death experiences?" "How were you disciplined as a child?" "Have you had any unusual illnesses or injuries?" "Were you ever raped or sexually molested?" Without specific questions, trauma disorder symptoms may be misidentified. None of the symptoms in the *DSM-III-R* criteria for PTSD are unique to that disorder (Domash & Sparr, 1982) and the PTSD patient often has concurrent illness, in which case the PTSD is often overlooked (Behar, 1984; Benedikt & Kolb, 1986; Sierles et al., 1983).

Resistance to discussing the trauma itself is not necessarily a sign of evasiveness. On the contrary, a flat, matter-of-fact report of a painful and terrifying story should lead the clinician to consider diagnoses that account for flattened affect, such as histrionic or schizoid personality disorders. I have heard several persons claiming to have been traumatized Vietnam veterans tell horrid stories without affect. Evasiveness or minimization of trauma events may reflect ego defenses, such as denial (not of facts, but of emotional impact), eye-witness confusion (E. Loftus & T. Loftus, 1980), or fear of reawakening or exacerbating PTSD symptoms. Horowitz (1985), in a letter poignantly titled "The Unreal Real and the Really Unreal," describes the confusing weave of fantasy and reality related to trauma events, where facts become dreams and obsessive fantasy to the extent that the survivor can no longer make a clear distinction. Trauma events are to the victims anomalous, once-in-a-lifetime events, such as the tornado that destroys the family home. If the trauma event is symbolic of the survivor's own psychology (e.g., the tornado survivor hated the house and wanted to move), then the trauma takes on special meaning. In another example, a man who hated his mother as a soldier witnessed a mother who was holding her child have her throat cut by another soldier. The murderer's commander (a Korean) immediately shot and killed the soldier. The witness who hated his mother never discussed the event with anyone in authority. It remained a memory that happened to express his own psychological problem.

Dissociation (Spiegel, 1984), as well as amnesia (Russell & Nathan, 1946; Schacter, 1986), presents problems for the survivor's recall of traumatic events. Trauma may happen under extraordinary conditions, eliciting fear and excitement. It may occur while one is under the mind-altering influence of chemicals (e.g., the drunken or drugged driver who loses control of a vehicle). Such conditions lead to confusion in reporting details. Terr (1983) has documented time distortions in the recall of trauma events in both child and adult survivors.

Obtaining objective evidence that a traumatic event has occurred is necessary, but frequently difficult. For the man who witnessed the murder of the mother, the only verification that could be obtained was his military records, which certified that he was in combat where he claimed to have seen the murder. Unfortunately, many violent crimes happen in isolation (Burgess & Holmstrom, 1979) and events may be traumatic because the survivor was isolated or abandoned, as with accidents in which one survives when others have died. In such cases, as well as in cases in which war veterans claim to have been traumatized serving outside their documented roles, it is crucial that the clinician obtain collateral reports describing the patient's adjustment before and after the event. Having a spouse, close relatives, or friends complete a clinical symptom checklist (Horowitz, Welner, & Alverez, 1979) or respond to a structured interview has been useful in identifying trauma symptoms. Checklists are especially helpful with alexithymic clients who are unable to articulate emotions. Krystal (1979) found that alexithymia (the inability to say how one feels) was a symptom often linked to psychic trauma.

Within reasonable limits, clinicians should not put themselves in a position of judging whether described events warrant the term "traumatic." Rather, the clinician should endeavor to view the event through the eyes of the survivor. Several authors have observed that the essence of psychic trauma lies in the meaning the experience has for the survivor (Hendin et al., 1981; Terr, 1979; Titchener, 1970). For instance, an individual's perception of whether an event is life-threatening does not depend on objective reality. The perspective of a child might differ from that of an adult. A person who was abused as a child and then traumatized again as an adult will attach additional meaning to the second traumatic event. If one were ever shot at, the unanticipated sight of a gun might elicit life-threatening emotions not experienced by other observers. The person who survives when others die also attaches special meaning to the trauma (Niederland, 1968, 1981). One who is traumatized after a prolonged period of exhaustion or starvation will have less energy with which to cope with the threat (Hocking, 1970). The person who is traumatized by repeated abuse and confinement attaches idiosyncratic meaning that the clinician must consider in arriving at an evaluation. Thus, the evaluation must consider the age, mental status, and especially the history of the survivor in relation to the traumatic event. Only then can the symptoms begin to make sense.

Once the traumatic event has been determined, the issue of simulated PTSD arises: (a) when symptoms are presented that are extreme or rare, or are inconsistent with the disorder (e.g., symptom-specific paralysis was more commonly reported after World War I [Kardiner, 1941] than today); (b) when there is secondary gain, especially when criminal charges or monetary claims are involved; and (c) when the known facts relating to the traumatic events contradict the patient's report, or when the patient's report of facts is internally inconsistent and self-contradictory.

Personality and cultural characteristics, such as antisocial or histrionic personality disorder or drug abuse (Sierles, 1984), cannot be a disqualification for the diagnosis of PTSD. Such variables characterize the very groups that are at high risk for trauma (Centers for Disease Control, 1987). Raifman (1983, p. 124n) asks if all persons with premorbid antisocial personality should be excluded as "unsuitable" for the diagnosis of PTSD, although it is unclear whether he recommends such action. Atkinson et al. (1982) appear to go too far in the other direction when they state, "We advise [Veterans Administration] examiners that if violence, disturbed relationships, and alcohol and drug problems are not found together with more fundamental features and symptoms of post traumatic stress disorder, this diagnosis is not to be made" (p. 1120).

Spiro (1968) writes that "malingering should only be diagnosed in the absence of psychiatric illness and the presence of behavior appropriately adaptive to a clear-cut long-term goal" (p. 569). Differential diagnosis (to liberally paraphrase Phillips et al., 1983, pp. 423-424) separates factitious from malingered from real or exaggerated PTSD. The first issue is to establish whether a reported symptom is factitious. This entails the discovery that the patient is lying (e.g., the proverbial insurance detective who catches the blind claimant reading). The second step is to determine whether a given factitious symptom is voluntary. If a factitious symptom is involuntary, another *DSM-III-R* diagnosis is used (viz. conversion disorder, somatoform pain disorder, or somatization disorder, etc.). If the symptom is voluntary, a diagnosis of factitious disorder or malingering is appropriate. The third step in the diagnostic process is to determine the client's goal in presenting the voluntarily produced symptom. If the client's goal is to become a patient for the sake of being a patient, then the diagnosis is factitious disorder.

CONCURRENT DISORDERS

The person who is prepsychotic or schizophrenic is quite vulnerable to psychic trauma. Jefferies (1977) argues that psychosis per se is traumatic, and, further, "that the consequent effects on one's self-esteem and ego identity may be such as to precipitate a traumatic neurosis" (p. 199). One man I recently evaluated, who appeared to have been accurately diagnosed as schizophrenic by several clinicians, described the traumatic impact of seeing a sexually mutilated corpse hanging from a tree in Vietnam, while on a brief shore-party detail from a cargo ship. The sight of the corpse alone, given this man's obsessional, psychotic process, was sufficient to be classified as a traumatic stressor.

Evaluations of persons who were traumatized years previously require careful assessment of the period immediately following the identified traumatic event (Burke et al., 1982). Acute PTSD symptoms, related to the avoidance and re-experiencing of the trauma, are often unaffected by psychological sophistication that may be subsequently acquired by the victim from advocates, counselors, or lawyers. The VA separates this "social work" phase of the evaluation process to precede the "psychiatric" evaluation and diagnosis (Atkinson et al., 1982), although such collateral research is often crucial to the diagnostic process.

An adult with a diagnosis of personality disorder has a high likelihood of having experienced trauma in childhood and is thus susceptible to extreme symptoms if traumatized a second time (Blumberg, 1979; Damlouji & Ferguson, 1985; Luisada, Peele, & Pittard, 1974). Krystal (1967), among others, has observed that the effects of trauma are cumulative. Titchener and Kapp (1976) have described permanent "character change" in trauma survivors where loss of community is involved.

The one symptom that is present in many cases of factitious PTSD is narcissism, with a sense of self-importance attached to the meaning of the trauma event or its impact. While trauma may be real in the history of someone with personality disorder, such persons are also at risk for identity confusions and may attach themselves to salient events in the press or current fads in the popular culture. I have encountered several men who claimed to have been traumatized in Vietnam, but on further investigation proved to be lying or imagining their traumas. Some were not veterans at all; others, although veterans, had never served in Vietnam, or had served there in a noncombatant capacity. Several of these men had demanding, sometimes abusive and dominating fathers, who were former military men. Others had childhoods that were extremely disrupted so that a solid identity never formed. Secondary gain was not always obvious in their current situation. Some appeared only to wish to be a part of the Vietnam veteran burgeoning "brotherhood" and joined rap sessions. Indeed, the gain seems not so much involved in explaining the crime to others, or some other immediate benefit, as in establishing a romantic identity. Post-traumatic stress disorder conveniently explains the symptoms of personality disorder, such as alienation and emotional lability, by attributing the problems to an extraordinary event. Such persons may create a fiction that they come to believe (i.e., a pseudologia fantastica) similar to that described by Phillips et al. (1983) in patients with factitious grief.

Any time one identifies trauma in childhood, or redefines the behavior of an influential family member as disturbed, one is capable of explaining much of one's personality development. Looking at development from a perspective of trauma may help to understand one's adult reactions to events, but unless the understanding is accompanied by some sort of prophylaxis, little more than understanding is achieved. For example, if one identifies a severe illness in early childhood that required prolonged hospitalization and removal from parents, subsequent depressions may be understood as related to feelings of abandonment. Such an understanding may explain one's over-reaction to a spouse's neglect. However, unless one can anticipate the cues relating to the original stressor, one has done little in terms of treatment.

EXAGGERATING
POST-TRAUMATIC STRESS DISORDER

Given the fact that a trauma did occur, an issue that faces the evaluator is whether the client is exaggerating the symptoms of trauma disorder. For example, a traumatized client may have originally experienced PTSD symptoms that have since remitted, but are presented to the evaluator as if they are current. Krystal (1967) comments on this issue, referring to compensation hearings of survivors of nazi death camps: "I saw many who did not so much want the money for itself as they did as a sign of recognition of the wrongs which were done . . . They wanted some modicum of justice" (p. 99). I have heard this sentiment voiced repeatedly by accident victims and by Vietnam veterans regarding their VA claims.

Exaggerating PTSD symptoms may thus be motivated by a survivor's lack of faith that the evaluation process will correctly identify the meaning of the trauma that the survivor has experienced. There is also the need to be recognized for the worst that one has suffered, which may have been during the acute phase of recovery, and a more severe process than one is undergoing during the evaluation period. The issue remains, however, for the evaluator to assess accurately the current adjustment of the trauma survivor.

There are several caveats here. The first concerns the episodic nature of post-traumatic stress disorder and the fact that, unlike most other psychiatric disorders, PTSD may have sudden onset and extreme symptoms, with almost complete remission (Rogers, 1986, p. 68).

The second caveat concerns the examiner who is being paid by the compensating agency, as for example, the VA evaluator who is contracting with the federal government. The question is not just one of conflict of interest, but may include more subtle issues of the evaluator's beliefs and values (Atkinson et al., 1982). Another example of this conflict occurred in Vietnam when mental health professionals were given more favorable evaluations according to the number of troops they returned to their units, and were rated negatively according to the number of troops sent out of Vietnam for treatment.

A third caveat concerns the problem of denial by professionals that trauma events can be permanently debilitating or life-altering (Krystal, 1967, p. 61; Titchener, 1970). Clinicians hesitate to predict permanent disability for a psychological disorder, yet massive or repeated traumas appear to have effects that are lifelong. In a society in which trauma is so pervasive, from the sexual abuse and traumatic discipline of children, to random stress, violence, rape, and domestic battering, as well as industrial accidents (Lopez-Ibor et al., 1985; Schottenfeld & Cullen, 1985), natural disasters, persecution, and discretionary wars, PTSD has become both a social and a clinical issue.

Kardiner wrote of this prophetically in 1941 when he described the resolution of "all other social issues" depending on our understanding of "traumatic neurosis." He predicted that traumatic neurosis would become "one of the commonest neurotic disturbances in the world" (Kardiner, 1941, p. v). The issue, for instance, of governmental budgeting for victim compensation and the extended and episodically required treatment of war trauma survivors is politically controversial. The controversy contributes to the ambivalence of professionals who must work within the constraints of institutional budget restrictions.

The reverse of this is the problem in which the term "trauma" is at risk of becoming as commonly used in our lexicon as the word "stress." People describe themselves as traumatized by vulgar language or minor accidents. The word "trauma" was frequently used by those commenting on the millions in the U.S. who watched the space shuttle explosion on television. While respecting our clients, we must adhere to the accepted clinical nosological definition of post-traumatic stress disorder. As Raifman (1983, p. 129) points out, we need to work toward an operational definition of "outside the range of common human experience."

EVALUATION PROBLEMS

It confounds the work of forensic evaluators when inconsistent and extreme symptoms are reported by trauma survivors as a reaction to the emotional disruption of anticipating and participating in clinical or forensic evaluation. One should not underestimate the anxiety that is generated in a trauma survivor by a clinical evaluation. Nightmares, for instance, are experienced by many survivors years after the traumatic event and can be renewed by clinical interviews. Van der Kolk et al. (1984) found that 59% of 199 sampled Vietnam veterans and 32% of 529 World War II and Korean War veterans experienced frequent nightmares. For the Vietnam veteran sample, "frequent" meant more than once a month. Some survivors define nightmares idiosyncratically and include semiconscious reverie connected with falling asleep and awakening. Others describe nightmares as any dream of a negative cast. Hartmann (1984) provides a reasonable lay definition of nightmares as "waking up from sleep terrified (without an external cause) or something from inside that awakens a person with a scared feeling" (p. 10). Such a definition, as Hartmann acknowledges, does not separate the nightmare from the Stage Four night terrors, which are usually imageless, but, because both are common in trauma survivors, the distinction is academic.

Flashbacks, similarly, are poorly defined. One must remember that PTSD is of the hysteria family (Hyler & Spitzer, 1978) and many trauma survivors, particularly those who were traumatized while their personalities were forming, tend to compartmentalize emotions. This tendency contributes to a variety of flashback phenomena. Some trauma survivors describe flashbacks as intense memories, while others describe dissociative experiences in which amnesic acting out of the trauma experience occurs (Blank, 1981). Drug and alcohol abuse contribute not only to the prolongation of trauma recovery, but also to the likelihood of flashback phenomena (Behar, 1984). The more the survivor is able to compartmentalize the trauma memory, the more the flashback will be unconscious and dissociative. In one case in my experience, a Vietnam army veteran burned down his house after a drunken argument with his wife, only to rescue his wife from the fire. He had been virtually asymptomatic for 15 years following the war, during which he had participated in the burning of a Vietnamese village. He had never told anyone of the event, and only told me while in an altered state of consciousness in the hospital room immediately after the blaze. Two weeks later, he had no recollection of telling the story, although when reminded, he related the event in sparse detail.

Raifman (1983) argues logically that the question of malingering is best left to a jury to decide and that "the use of mental health professionals' evaluations to detect malingering creates more problems than it solves . . ." (p. 126n). Albeit problematic, the use of nonspecific, subtle questioning of both the trauma survivor and intimate collaterals over several weeks provides the most reliable separation of real from exaggerated or malingered PTSD. Unfortunately, many institutions allow only a short time (sometimes an hour or less; Atkinson et al., 1982) for a diagnostic claim interview. Such a brief period may be appropriate for a trauma survivor who is articulate and specific, but for many, especially those who are culturally or ethnically different from the evaluator, several hour-long interviews are warranted in order to understand the survivor's language and personality style and thus assess the impact of the trauma. That understanding includes what Raifman (1983) refers to as the "symptom-specific" behavior (p. 122), such as anniversary reactions (Cavenar, Nash, & Maltbie, 1978) and over-reactive affect (Krystal, 1978, p. 88).

I once evaluated a woman who had been in a frightening motor vehicle accident in which the car in which she was a passenger went out of control on an elevated bridge and crashed through a guard rail and into a house. She was an obese, middle-aged Puerto Rican woman who had previously been treated with antipsychotic medication for auditory hallucinations. She had also been involved in a prior accident claim. She had a histrionic style and spoke in jargon and with an unusual accent. She had been treated cavalierly by emergency personnel at the scene, driven to a hospital emergency room in a van, and released with a cursory examination. The woman was demanding and flirtatious, and responded to my questions with obscure, rambling, and seemingly loose associations. I, as a White, male, middle-class PhD in the Pacific Northwest, had to proceed very cautiously to identify the symptoms of PTSD. She had had a potentially traumatic experience. She thought she was going to die. She experienced symptom-specific anxieties and fears, sleep disturbance, and nightmares. She also experienced exaggerated panic and psychotic symptoms when she thought she was going to be abandoned by her family and ignored by professionals. Although she had worked steadily prior to the accident, it had been at a menial job and she showed no regret at not returning to work. This woman had a variety of psychiatric evaluations and a number of diagnoses both before and after the accident. At least one evaluation was clearly prejudiced against her, and yet there was no question in my mind, after I spent several hours with her, that she was experiencing PTSD in addition to her personality disorder.

Questions regarding untoward, highly emotional symptoms specific to a stressful event must be phrased with an understanding of the survivor's cultural style and personality. When the evaluator is one of several, the relationship with the client needs to be established before diagnostic clarity can be achieved. It is only in the context of the relationship that rehearsed or disguised and guarded information can be identified. The work of Kolb (1987) and others cited in his provocative 1987 review of the physiology of PTSD illustrates the panic-like arousal that is usually symptom specific to the trauma. In such cases as Kolb describes, imagery recalling the trauma scene, such as the sounds of the battlefield or the automobile crash, evoke autonomic responses appropriate for the emergency demanded by the trauma. Aggressive, time-constrained interviewing that is insensitive to such arousal, and, indeed, may even seek to elicit such arousal, can worsen the condition of the trauma disorder. It is inappropriate, therefore, to subject a client to a deliberate elicitation of such an arousal state solely for the sake of gathering forensic evidence.

PSYCHOMETRIC EVALUATION

Rogers (1986) asserts that "abundant evidence indicates that individuals are aware of personality characteristics they reveal in projective testing" (p. 136). It is reasonable to assume that many people who are creative enough to sham PTSD can produce relevant Rorschach imagery, though perhaps not the "negative symptoms" of PTSD (e.g., imagery relating to barrier penetration). However, I have found the Rorschach helpful in identifying trauma in very anxious clients who employed denial in repressing trauma experiences or the emotional impact of traumatogenic events.

The Minnesota Multiphasic Personality Inventory (MMPI) offers more promise in detecting persons who exaggerate symptoms. Rogers (1986) recommends the MMPI F-K index, and the so-called "subtle-obvious" elevations (pp. 142-146). Gough (1950) found that an F-K raw score differential greater than 16 identified two-thirds of the subjects who were faking bad. An F-K raw score cutoff of 7 is recommended to identify 95% of the persons with authentic symptoms. In many forensic situations, however, even a 5% risk of error is too great. Fairbank, McCaffrey, & Keane (1985) suggest that an F-scale T-score above 88 identifies fabricators. Buckhart, Christian, and Gynther (1978) found that, when a subject faked good, MMPI subtle items increased and obvious items decreased, whereas the reverse was true when a subject faked bad (i.e., subtle items decreased but obvious items increased). Buckhart et al. identified this as a paradox, although it may be a reflection of what Flicker (1956) called the "symptom" of malingering, which is a paradox.

149

The paradox of the malingering "symptom" is this: If malingering must be diagnosed only in the absence of relevant symptoms, then the intent of pretending suffering to avoid work or responsibility for criminal acts cannot be seen as symptomatic of a clinical disorder. One cannot argue that a client is malingering because he or she is depressed and anhedonic, or because the client has an antisocial personality and is in conflict with established authority. Thus, to be logically consistent, the client may malinger if he or she has a personality disorder, so long as the personality disorder is not the cause of the malingering. However, if the disorder is involved in generating the motivation to lie - for instance, if the lying is compulsive - then a diagnosis other than malingering must be made. In cases of PTSD, work anhedonia is a symptom that may lead to erratic job history and secondary conflicts regarding the motives for claiming benefits.

Persons with combat-related PTSD commonly show elevations on clinical scales of the MMPI (Keane, Malloy, & Fairbank, 1984). The 2-8 or 8-2 profile is frequently seen, reflecting the depression and alienation of having painful images and emotions that are difficult to communicate. For such clients, a high F-K index is not uncommon. I have treated clients who were extremely anxious and angry, who abused drugs and alcohol since their initial traumas, and who scored with an F-scale above 90 (T-score). Such persons who are anxious about their symptoms will have profiles with obvious well over subtle, and yet have well-documented trauma experiences with symptoms prolonged and exacerbated by substance abuse and personality style. This is essentially the sort of client likely to be labeled as "fake bad" or malingering. Rogers' (1986) caveat is worth respecting: "No MMPI profile should be used to indicate directly responsibility or non-responsibility" (p. 144) for a crime. Nor should the MMPI be used as the sole evaluation method. Rogers states further (p. 74) that malingering should be diagnosed only after "numerous and convincing examples" are identified. Gough (1950), in his early work on the MMPI, states that scores on L, F, and K scales "have relevance to the personality structure of the test taker as well as to the reliability and meaningfulness of his [sic] test protocol, per se" (p. 408).

There is a relative cost when a clinician makes a diagnostic error, and usually the cost of error in forensic or claims hearings is significant. The clinical evaluator must consider the tendency to blame the survivors for carelessness or poor judgment, or wishing their traumas were not so pervasive or chronic. The issue of rewarding a malingerer (false positive) versus denying a trauma survivor (false negative) is not just one of justice, but also of good professional practice, since appropriate treatment often follows accurate recognition and diagnosis of the disorder.

SUMMARY

Post-traumatic stress disorder is a diagnosis that is seldom made with clarity when secondary gain is suggested. Standard forensic methods must be used with caution. In most cases, a series of interviews spanning several appointments is preferable to the intense, brief consultation. Where possible, in addition to the clinical interview, the evidence should include use of the MMPI and data from pertinent collaterals, preferably using a somewhat structured interview, symptoms checklist, or "impact of events" scale. Evidence for malingering should be clear and unassailable before the diagnosis is made. The existence of PTSD in a claimant does not necessarily indicate that the disorder is caused by the trauma event in question. Symptoms specific to the trauma event should be identified in cases of persons who have survived multiple traumas.

Factitious PTSD is likely to increase in frequency with the increasing notoriety of the diagnosis. It is evident that PTSD is attractive to those with personality disorders, others with poorly formed identities, and those wishing to take on the role of the survivor seeking justice. Because psychic trauma is so common in our society, it is considered a social problem.

Emmett Early, PhD, is a clinical psychologist in private practice in Seattle, Washington. He is a frequent lecturer on the subject of post-traumatic stress disorder and on Jungian theoretical approaches to the trauma complex. He began his interest in post-traumatic stress disorder when he became involved in the Veterans Administration Vets Center outreach program in 1979. Although his full-time private practice is a general adult analytic practice, he maintains a special interest in trauma disorder. He is a clinical consultant for Vietnam veteran readjustment problems with the

Washington State Department of Veterans Affairs, and has conducted long-term psychotherapy groups for combat veterans for the past 7 years. Dr. Early may be contacted at 4719 University Way, N.E., #206, Seattle, WA 98105.

REFERENCES

Akhtar, S. (1984). The syndrome of identity diffusion. *American Journal of Psychiatry, 141,* 1381-1385.

American Psychiatric Association. (1987). *Diagnostic and Statistical Manual of Mental Disorders* (3rd ed., rev.). Washington, DC: Author.

Atkinson, R., Henderson, R., & Sparr, L. (1982). Assessment of Viet Nam veterans for posttraumatic stress disorder in Veterans Administration disability claims. *American Journal of Psychiatry, 139,* 1118-1121.

Behar, D. (1984). Confirmation of concurrent illnesses in post traumatic stress disorder. *American Journal of Psychiatry, 141,* 1310.

Benedikt, R., & Kolb, L. (1986). Preliminary findings on chronic pain and post traumatic stress disorder. *American Journal of Psychiatry, 143,* 908-910.

Blank, A. (1981 rev.). *The Unconscious Flashback to the War in Vietnam Veterans: Clinical Mystery, Legal Defense, and Community Problem.* Paper presented at the American Psychological Association Annual Meeting, Montreal, Quebec, Canada. (Originally 1980)

Blumberg, M. (1979). Character disorders in traumatized and handicapped children. *American Journal of Psychotherapy, 33,* 201-213.

Buckhart, B., Christian, W., & Gynther, M. (1978). Item subtlety and faking on the MMPI: A paradoxical relationship. *Journal of Personality Assessment, 42,* 76-80.

Burgess, A., & Holmstrom, L. (1979). *Rape, Crisis and Recovery.* Bowie, MD: R. J. Brady Co.

Burke, J., Borus, J., Millstein, K., & Beasley, M. (1982). Changes in children's behavior after a natural disaster. *American Journal of Psychiatry, 139,* 1010-1014.

Cavenar, J., Nash, J., & Maltbie, A. (1978). Anniversary reactions presenting as physical complaints. *Journal of Clinical Psychiatry, 39,* 369-374.

Centers for Disease Control. (1987). Post service mortality among Vietnam veterans: The Centers for Disease Control Vietnam experience study. *Journal of the American Medical Association, 257,* 790-795.

Cohen, J. (1981). Theories of narcissism and trauma. *American Journal of Psychotherapy, 35,* 93-100.

Damlouji, N., & Ferguson, J. (1985). Three cases of post traumatic anorexia nervosa. *American Journal of Psychiatry, 142,* 362-363.

Diamond, B. (1971). Failures of identification and sociopathic behavior. In S. S. Furst (Ed.), *Sanctions for Evil* (pp. 125-135). Boston, MA: Beacon Press.

Domash, M., & Sparr, L. (1982). Post traumatic stress disorder masquerading as paranoid schizophrenia: Case report. *Military Medicine, 147,* 772-774.

Early, E. (1984). On confronting the Vietnam veteran. *American Journal of Psychiatry, 141,* 472-473.

Erlinder, C. (1983). Post traumatic stress disorder, Vietnam veterans and the law: A challenge to effective representation. *Behavior Sciences and the Law, 1,* 25-50.

Fairbank, J., McCaffrey, R., & Keane, T. (1985). Psychometric detection of fabricated symptoms of PTSD. *American Journal of Psychiatry, 142,* 501-503.

Flicker, D. (1956). Malingering--A symptom. *Journal of Nervous and Mental Disease, 1,* 23-31.

Goodwin, J. (Undated). *Continuing Readjustment Problems among Vietnam Veterans.* Cincinnati, OH: Disabled American Veterans.

Gough, H. (1950). The F-K dissimulation index for the Minnesota Multiphasic Personality Inventory. *Journal of Consulting Psychology, 14,* 408-413.

Hartmann, E. (1984). *The Nightmare: The Psychology and Biology of Terrifying Dreams.* New York: Basic Books.

Hefez, A., Metz, L., & Lavie, P. (1987). Long term effects of extreme situational stress on sleep and dreaming. *American Journal of Psychiatry, 144,* 344-347.

Hendin, H., Pollinger, A., Singer, P., & Ulman, R. (1981). Meanings of combat and the development of PTSD. *American Journal of Psychiatry, 138,* 1490-1493.

Hocking, F. (1970). Extreme environmental stress and its significance for psychopathology. *American Journal of Psychotherapy, 24,* 4-26.

Horowitz, M. (1985). The unreal real and the really unreal. *American Journal of Psychiatry, 142,* 1131.

Horowitz, M., Welner, N., & Alverez, W. (1979). Impact of events scale: A measure of subjective stress. *Psychological Medicine, 41,* 209-318.

Hyler, S., & Spitzer, R. (1978). Hysteria split asunder. *American Journal of Psychiatry, 135,* 1500-1504.

Jefferies, J. (1977). The trauma of being psychotic. *Canadian Psychiatric Association Journal, 22,* 199-205.

Kardiner, A. (1941). *The Traumatic Neuroses of War.* New York: Harper & Bros.

Keane, T., Malloy, P., & Fairbank, J. (1984). Empirical development of an MMPI subscale for the assessment of combat related post traumatic stress disorder. *Journal of Consulting and Clinical Psychology, 52,* 888-891.

Kolb, L. (1987). A neuropsychological hypothesis explaining post traumatic stress disorders. *American Journal of Psychiatry, 144,* 989-995.

Krystal, H. (1967). *Massive Psychic Trauma.* New York: International Universities Press.

Krystal, H. (1978). Trauma and affects. *Psychoanalytic Study of the Child, 33,* 81-116.

Krystal, H. (1979). Alexithymia and psychotherapy. *American Journal of Psychotherapy, 33,* 17-31.

LaGuardia, R., Smith, G., Francois, R., & Bachman, L. (1983). Incidence of delayed stress disorder among Vietnam era veterans: The effect of priming on response set. *American Journal of Orthopsychiatry, 53,* 18-26.

Lavie, P., Hefez, A., Halperin, G., & Enoch, D. (1979). Long term effects of traumatic war-related events on sleep. *American Journal of Psychiatry, 136,* 175-178.

Loftus, E., & Loftus, T. (1980). On the impermanence of stored information in the human brain. *American Psychologist, 35,* 409-420.

Lopez-Ibor, J., Soria, J., Canas, R., & Rodriguez-Gamazo, M. (1985). Psychopathological aspects of the toxic oil syndrome catastrophe. *British Journal of Psychiatry, 147,* 352-365.

Luisada, P., Peele, R., & Pittard, E. (1974). The hysterical personality in men. *American Journal of Psychiatry, 131,* 518-522.

Mayfield, D., & Fowler, D. (1969). Combat plus 20 years: The effect of previous combat experience on psychiatric patients. *Military Medicine, 134,* 13-48.

Niederland, W. (1968). Clinical observations on the survivor syndrome. *International Journal of Psychoanalysis, 49,* 313-315.

Niederland, W. (1981). The survivor syndrome: Further observations and dimensions. *Journal of the American Psychoanalytic Association, 29,* 413-425.

Phillips, M., Ward, N., & Ries, R. (1983). Factitious mourning: Painless patienthood. *American Journal of Psychiatry, 140,* 420-425.

Raifman, L. (1983). Problems of diagnosis and legal causation in courtroom use of post traumatic stress disorder. *Behavior Science and the Law, 1,* 115-130.

Resnick, P. (1984). The detection of malingered mental illness. *Behavior Science and the Law, 2,* 21-38.

Rogers, R. (1986). *Conducting Insanity Evaluations.* New York: Van Nostrand Reinhold.

Russell, W., & Nathan, P. (1946). Traumatic amnesia. *Brain, 69,* 280-300.

Schacter, D. (1986). Amnesia and crime: How much do we really know? *American Psychologist, 41,* 286-295.

Schottenfeld, R., & Cullen, M. (1985). Occupation-induced post traumatic stress disorders. *American Journal of Psychiatry, 142,* 198-202.

Scurfield, R., & Blank, A. (1986). A guide to obtaining a military history from Vietnam veterans. In S. M. Sonnenberg, A. S. Blank, & J. M. Talbott (Eds.), *The Trauma of War* (pp. 265-290). Washington, DC: American Psychiatric Press.

Sierles, F. (1984). Correlates of malingering. *Behavior Sciences and the Law, 2,* 113-118.

Sierles, F. S., Chen, J. J., McFarland, R. E., & Taylor, M. A. (1983). Post traumatic stress disorder and concurrent psychiatric illness: A preliminary report. *American Journal of Psychiatry, 140,* 1177-1179.

Solomon, Z., Garb, R., Bleich, A., & Grupper, D. (1987). Reactivation of combat-related post traumatic stress disorder. *American Journal of Psychiatry, 144,* 51-55.

Sparr, L., & Pankratz, L. (1983). Factitious post traumatic stress disorder. *American Journal of Psychiatry, 140,* 1016-1019.

Spiegel, D. (1984). Multiple personality as post traumatic stress disorder. *Psychiatric Clinics of North America, 7,* 101-110.

Spiro, H. (1968). Chronic factitious illness: Münchausen's syndrome. *Archives of General Psychiatry, 18,* 569-579.

Stern, G. (1976). *The Buffalo Creek Disaster.* New York: Random House.

Symonds, M. (1980). The "second injury" to victims [Special issue]. *Evaluation and Change,* pp. 36-38.

Terr, L. (1979). Children of Chowchilla: A study of psychic trauma. *Psychoanalytic Study of the Child, 34,* 547-623.

Terr, L. (1983). Time sense following psychic trauma: Clinical study of 10 adults and 20 children. *American Journal of Orthopsychiatry, 53,* 244-261.

Titchener, J. (1970). Management and study of psychological response to trauma. *Journal of Trauma, 10,* 974-980.

Titchener, J., & Kapp, F. (1976). Family and character change at Buffalo Creek. *American Journal of Psychiatry, 133,* 295-299.

van der Kolk, B., Blitz, R., Burr, W., Sherry, S., & Hartmann, E. (1984). Nightmares and trauma: A comparison of nightmares after combat with lifelong nightmares in veterans. *American Journal of Psychiatry, 141,* 187-190.

Van Dyke, C., Zilberg, N., & McKinnon, J. (1985). Post traumatic stress disorder: A thirty year delay in a World War Two veteran. *American Journal of Psychiatry, 142,* 1070-1073.

Wilmer, H. (1982). Vietnam and madness: Dreams of schizophrenic veterans. *The Journal of the American Academy of Psychoanalysis, 10,* 47-65.

7.

Forensic Issues in Post-Traumatic Stress Disorder

Herbert C. Modlin

Forensic psychiatry and psychology are professional subspecialties concerned with the overlapping areas and services of the legal and the mental health professions. A citizen may become a client of both the legal and medical social systems simultaneously if questions of mental functioning are relevant to a criminal or civil procedure in which the citizen is involved. When mental health professionals come into contact with the law through patients or former patients, they will encounter legal concepts, vocabulary, ethics, and societal functions strikingly different from those of their own disciplines.

This chapter will be limited to civil law issues directly related to persons with the diagnosis of post-traumatic stress disorder (PTSD) and will discuss tort law, personal injury, product liability, workers' compensation, proximate cause, predisposition, estimates of disability, and report writing. It will not cover such important general forensic topics as confidentiality and privilege, informed consent, malpractice claims, the differing roles and responsibilities of examining and treating clinicians, or the functions of expert witnesses in trials, hearings, and depositions. The main purpose here is to acquaint the uninitiated with legal vocabulary, concepts, and attitudes relating to the involvement of PTSD patients in litigation.

PERSONAL INJURY SUITS

The law of torts is concerned with civil rather than criminal offenses. Prosser (1971) begins his classical treatise on torts observing that a really satisfactory definition of a tort has yet to be found, and then illuminates the subject through a thousand pages. Citizens are expected to assume certain civic duties in relation to other citizens, and if they violate those responsibilities, they become potential targets for lawsuits.

The law of torts includes a number of possible actions against a presumed perpetrator based on a charge of trespass, negligence, slander, plagiarism, false representation (deceit), invasion of privacy, or malicious persecution. One has a duty to see that one halts at the stop sign, prevents one's dog from biting the mail carrier, clears one's icy sidewalk, and refrains from spreading false rumors about an acquaintance, or taking snapshots of one's neighbor sunbathing unclad in her yard.

Personal injury suits commonly proceed within the aegis of the legal theory of negligence, that is, an unintentional breach of tort that damages a victim. If the harm is intentional, the perpetrator becomes liable to criminal prosecution, which, however, does not preclude a possible concurrent civil action for recovery of damages. To press a civil suit successfully, the plaintiff must assume the burden of proof and show that (a) a legal duty of care existed, (b) which the defendant fulfilled negligently, and (c) resulting in substantial damage to the plaintiff (Prosser, 1971).

If the attorney decides that his or her client's potential legal case has merit, that is, he or she can marshal good evidence to prove that the defendant is liable for the client's injuries, he or she will then call on the mental health clinician for a determination of damage to the plaintiff. That finding is crucial: If there is no damage, there is no suit, no matter how negligent the defendant's behavior. Therefore, the client's report and the testimony of the clinical expert may make or break the case.

Some personal injury claims invoke the concept of product liability, a new and rapidly developing branch of tort law. Manufacturers and retailers are being held liable in distributing products that may have deleterious effects on consumers. The mental health professional may hear of product liability with increasing frequency. The manufacturer has a duty to present a product free of potentially dangerous defects and to include with the product directions for its proper use and warnings about the consequences of misuse. The clinical syndromes in such cases will not vary from those precipitated by other kinds of accidents, although there could be some concomitant physical damage.

For example, consider the case of a man opening a bottle of soda. The bottle explodes, and the cap flies into his eye, permanently blinding it. He demonstrates symptoms of PTSD: tension and insomnia, and he dreams of being in an explosion. He becomes quite depressed, in addition, over the loss of his eye. On his attorney's advice, he sues the manufacturers of the bottle and cap, the manufacturer and distributor of the soda, and the retail store that sold the product.

WORKERS' COMPENSATION CLAIMS

Workers' compensation law emerged at the turn of the century in the wake of the Industrial Revolution. As populations shifted from farm to factory, the incidence of accidental injuries became alarming. The law evolved to place the costs of occupational disability on the employer regardless of fault or negligence on either side, and thus to free claims from litigation. Neither worker nor employer had to retain an attorney and courts were relieved of large workloads. Under the present laws in all 50 states, awards granted by Workers' Compensation Commissions are for lost wages and medical expenses, and an additional award for loss of life. All employers carry insurance and, if there is any problem, the worker must negotiate with an insurance company, not the employer.

In the mental health field, the enactment of the law is quite uneven because many insurance companies take a conservative position in doling out money for seemingly intangible and frequently suspect claims of mental and emotional damage. Many state laws support this position concerning so "nebulous" a concept as neurosis and require evidence of physical injury to validate a claim of traumatic neurosis. The phrase "traumatic neurosis" is the universal label used in the law, although in the past few years, PTSD has appeared in some commission and court documents (Modlin, 1983). Still, PTSD must be shown to have derived directly from physical damage. Consequently, most persons suffering from PTSD due to a frightening work-related accident are referred by attorneys to mental health professionals because the worker, often on advice from his or her union office, has had to consult an attorney for help with a recalcitrant insurance company.

Proper clinical evaluation of an injured worker may be complicated by environmental factors impinging on the plaintiff that are seldom explored in workers' compensation suits. These include the "war" between union and management, a cynical plant medical department, a skeptical insurance company, and an impersonal compensation commission. There may be unfortunate shifts in family dynamics as the disabled head-of-household loses status at home (Modlin, 1986). The factor of secondary gain may loom large, although that should not negate the claim since it is, by definition, unconsciously determined. The testifying clinician should explain and differentiate secondary gain from such conscious attitudes as revenge or cupidity.

PROXIMATE CAUSE

The law requires that the presumed cause of the plaintiff's (claimant's) disability be directly related to the disability within a reasonable time frame. The law also cautions that there be no other important determinants that are not the responsibility of the defendant. Among the common precipitants of PTSD are unexpected frightening events such as highway accidents, work-related accidents, defects in commercial products, assault, rape, natural disasters, war experiences, and terrorist activities. Such factors or occurrences can attributively be connected to the onset of PTSD.

In an appropriate case, the clinician should be prepared to explain that although the patient was experiencing one or more other life stressors at the time (failing marriage, loss of job, death of a child), the proximate cause of the PTSD had to be the traumatizing accident. The clinician must also be prepared to explain, buttressed by literature citations, the onset of delayed PTSD 2 months after the accident. He or she may also need to state that the plaintiff's depression or generalized anxiety disorder (GAD), which continued after PTSD symptoms have largely subsided, are probably due to other factors. The issue of "proximate cause" is demonstrated in the following case example:

G.H. (17 years old) was walking with her parents past a store when an explosion occurred. A large plate-glass window erupted, breaking across her head. She developed a classical PTSD syndrome: nightmares of explosions; severe startle reaction to sudden noises; the typical anxiety, tension, insomnia, and concentration difficulty; and mild concern over her slightly scarred face. When evaluated 3 months after the accident, she was tense, depressed, and tearful. As the story unfolded, her present plight was found to be due, primarily, to guilt over sexual relations with a boyfriend and his obviously waning interest in her. The clinician informed the attorney that his client had 1 or 2 months of moderate disability from the PTSD precipitated by the accident, but it was not the proximate cause of her current untoward symptoms.

PREDISPOSITION

Behavioral scientists assume that life is a continuum, that the past is indeed prologue. Hereditary, congenital, and environmental influences determine, from conception onward, personality traits, ego weaknesses, and character strengths that the organism has available for coping with intrapsychic, interpersonal, environmental, and cultural stressors. Consequently, people vary in their susceptibility to breakdown. Onset of a mental illness depends as much on predisposition as on traumatic events. One aspect of tort and workers' compensation law often disconcerting to the mental health professional is that predisposition to mental breakdown is seldom considered relevant to the legal problem at hand.

The law of torts holds that the tortfeasor is equally liable whether his or her injurious offense caused the disability, activated a latent condition, or worsened a pre-existing condition. Justice Oliver Wendell Holmes (1909) once observed that the law is not just for the hale and hearty. He noted also that the law usually cannot take into account the infinite varieties of temperament, intellect, and education that make the character of a given act or reaction so different in different persons.

Tortfeasors take their victims as they find them; employers take their employees as they find them. This dictum may seem superficial or simplistic to the clinician, but the alternative would be impossible. Imagine the consternation of the mental health professional asked to determine the percentages of present disability in a given PTSD patient "caused" by childhood beatings, an alcoholic mother, a seductive stepbrother, a career setback, an unfaithful spouse, and the highway accident. The law in its wisdom largely chooses to settle plaintiff-defendant disputes in the here and now.

The "but for" theory is often invoked by plaintiff's attorneys and mental health professionals will be expected to respond to it. No matter what the history of the person, on the day of the accident he or she was employable, employed, financially solvent, engaged in an average marital relationship, enjoying a modicum of social activities, and PTSD symptom-free. Since the accident, he or she has been unemployed, in financial straits, straining the marriage with his or her behavior, in retreat from any social contacts, and suffering distressing and disabling symptoms. But for the accident, all these disasters would not have occurred. The traumatic event can be called a "last straw" phenomenon - but for the last straw, the camel might have plodded on indefinitely under his or her heavy burden.

DISABILITY

Trial attorneys are accustomed to working closely with physicians in arriving at an accurate estimate of a client's impairment or disability resulting from physical damage. The physician can state, after consulting an actuarial table, that the loss of a thumb merits a rating of 50% impairment of hand function; or the loss of an eye constitutes a 40% permanent impairment of vision. Attorneys should be disabused of possible hope for a similar precision from mental health professionals.

Mental health professionals are concerned chiefly with questions of disability in the person as a whole rather than impairment of a body part. We attempt to evaluate a patient as a biopsychosocial unit embedded in and interacting with an environment. Rarely can we estimate disability in other than general terms - mild, moderate, severe - and we should not feel defensive about this inexactitude.

In attempting a disability rating of PTSD patients, we need a clear understanding from the attorney about the legal questions to be addressed. For example, personal injury claims and workers' compensation claims have different disability standards. Also, does the attorney need a partial versus total or temporary versus permanent disability estimate? Workers' compensation law usually limits the disability issue to whether workers can return to their jobs, usually the ones they were performing when traumatized.

Workers' compensation is available for injury or illness arising in the course of employment, and only work capacity is considered in accepting or refusing a claim. As a result of the PTSD symptoms, the worker may have alienated his or her family by constant irritability, frustrated his or her spouse through sexual incapacity, strained friendships by social withdrawal, and relinquished avocational pleasures such as fishing, dancing, or reading. None of these components of a "good life" are relevant in workers' compensation claims. In a personal injury suit, all of these listed "losses" should be included in a clinical estimate of PTSD consequences.

One frequently necessary element of disability ratings that may generate dismay and reluctance on the part of mental health professionals is the law's need for them to prognosticate. The plaintiff's attorney will press clinicians for a statement on permanent disability or the duration of temporary disability, since that option will influence the monetary award requested. They are expected to contribute estimates of illness severity, treatability, length and cost of treatment, probable response to treatment, and likely extent of long-term disability.

G.H., a 13-year-old girl, suffered extensive burns from a car crash. In spite of several surgical repairs, disfiguring scars marred her face, neck, and one breast. She suffered a full-blown PTSD. To what extent will the consequences of the accident impair her future employability, marriageability, personality development, and general social acceptance? The law considers this a fair question, no matter how disconcerting to the clinician. The law's position is understandable: Litigants have only their day in court and the dispute must be entirely resolved. The plaintiff cannot reopen the case 5 years later if new disabilities surface or if treatment should be less than successful.

One aid in considering disability ratings is the manual published by the American Medical Association (1984).

Chapter 12, prepared by an expert committee of psychiatrists, presents guidelines for percentage ratings of the major components in mental and emotional functioning (Modlin, 1986). The text is couched in general terms, allowing leeway for the clinician in evaluating individual cases, but provides a useful frame of reference and helps the forensic clinician to exercise consistency from case to case.

REPORTS

Writers of reports presenting clinical data and conclusions from evaluation of a client should keep in mind the specific recipient of the report and the nature of its purpose. A communication to an attorney should differ from one sent to another mental health professional, a general medical practitioner, or a concerned relative. Since many PTSD sufferers are litigants, a report sent to an attorney or hearing judge should address clinical issues and responses to legal questions the writer anticipates might be asked.

Ordinarily in civil matters, including disputes under tort law, the report is not a confidential document from clinician to attorney. Most states have discovery provisions in civil cases, a departure from the rule in criminal law. Each side in the dispute can "discover" the opponent's data on request. The hope from this provision, borne out in practice, is that full disclosure on each side will encourage out-of-court settlement and obviate court trials. Consequently, it is important to recognize the potentially different levels of clinical understanding of persons who may read the report.

A clinician may be appalled to learn that the attorney allowed the client to read the report. Of course, that is not what the attorney did. From his or her perspective, the attorney provided the client with a document to keep the client abreast of progress in the litigation - an ethically defensible act in legal practice. But the clinician should be forewarned that the examinee might read the report. This does not mean that the clinician should be less than honest, but he or she can be appropriately tactful. If the diagnoses include "a mixed personality disorder with dependent, avoidant, and passive-aggressive features," so be it. The clinician need not belabor the point, as was done in one report on record where the litigant was described as a sad sack, an ineffectual bumbler, and a chronic parasite.

Reports should contain all the information necessary to support fully the clinical and legal opinions expressed. The reader should be able to comprehend how the conclusions were reached from the data in the body of the report. The writing should be intelligible to laypeople, and thus free of professional jargon. If the use of a technical term is necessary, the term should be clearly defined.

Presentation of a full report is one of the best devices available for keeping the clinician out of court. The attorney to whom the report is sent can often use it effectively in negotiation with his or her counterpart. He or she can say, approximately, "This is what my expert witness will testify to in court. Now, how about discussing settlement?"

Although, as explained previously, the report should contain all the data necessary to its purpose, it should contain only the necessary data. Legally irrelevant sensitive material should not be included - that is, the clinician need not, and probably should not, report everything he or she knows about the examinee; for example, earlier abortion or his adulterous affair have no bearing on the PTSD precipitated by a serious accident.

After preparing a report with reasonable consideration for protecting privacy, the mental health professional still may not find himself or herself safely out of the legal forest. An astute opposing counsel may have a subpoena served on the clinician requiring him or her to relinquish all records, including personal notes, psychotherapy progress records, raw psychological test data, statements of charges, correspondence, and so on. The clinician may have to comply and should not, under any circumstances, destroy any material; it not only would be illegal, but also dishonest. There are recourses: (a) immediately notify the patient's attorney of the opposing attorney's action; or (b) if in any doubt, consult one's own attorney or the one retained by one's professional organization.

Subpoenas are frequently prepared by court clerks and issued after a perfunctory glance and signature by a judge. It is quite possible for the litigant's attorney, with the clinician's help, to confer with the judge and get personal and irrelevant (to the legal case) material protected from disclosure.

CONCLUSION

To certain mental health professionals, participation in a forensic role is stimulating and thought provoking; others find it uncomfortable and confusing. The probability is, however, that most will practice some forensic psychiatry or psychology, even if involuntarily. In today's social, economic, and legal climate, clinicians cannot escape being drawn into forensic participation by patients, colleagues, institutions, and professional associations.

Herbert C. Modlin, PhD, received an honorable DSc degree from the University of Nebraska and did post-graduate work in psychiatry and neurology in Philadelphia, Boston, and Montreal (1940-1943). He was Chief of Neuropsychiatric Services at the Topeka VA Hospital in 1946-1949 and has been a staff member at the Menninger Clinic since 1949. He was a candidate at the Topeka Psychoanalytic Institute from 1947-1954. Dr. Modlin is board certified in psychiatry, neurology, and forensic psychiatry, and is a past President of the American Board of Forensic Psychiatry. He currently is a Professor of Forensic Psychiatry at the Menninger School of Psychiatry, and a visiting lecturer at the University of Kansas Medical School and Law School. His special interests include personal injury, stress response syndromes, and disaster syndromes, and he has numerous publications in these areas. Dr. Modlin can be reached at The Menninger Clinic, Box 829, Topeka, KS 66601-0829.

REFERENCES

American Medical Association. (1984). *Guides to the Evaluation of Permanent Impairment.* Chicago: Author.

Holmes, O., Jr. (1909). *The Common Law.* Boston: Little, Brown Co.

Modlin, H. (1983). Traumatic neuroses and other injuries. *Psychiatric Clinics of North America, 6,* 661-681.

Modlin, H. (1986). Compensation neurosis. *Bulletin of the American Academy of Psychiatry and Law, 14,* 263-272.

Prosser, W. (1971). *Handbook of the Law of Torts.* St. Paul, MN: West Publishing Co.

8.

Definitions, Procedures, and Guidelines for Expert Witnesses

Charles Z. Smith

THE THERAPIST AS WITNESS

The ordinary dictionary definition of "witness" includes (a) a person who attests to a fact or statement; (b) a person who saw, or can give a firsthand account of, something; (c) a person who testifies in court; (d) a person called upon to observe a transaction in order to testify concerning it if it is later held in question; and (e) something providing or serving as evidence (*Webster's New World Dictionary of the American Language*, 1960). Witnesses in legal proceedings may be identified before a complaint has been filed. Upon the happening of any event that is destined for litigation, any person who "saw, or can give a firsthand account of, something" is a potential witness.

Witnesses may be generally characterized as (a) witnesses for purposes of investigation or inquiry; (b) witnesses who are competent to testify in a legal proceeding based upon firsthand knowledge; and (c) "expert witnesses," who may be competent to testify in legal proceedings based upon their qualifications as "experts," and not necessarily because of firsthand knowledge.

Any person who observes an event is a potential witness to litigation involving that event. The witness may be voluntary or involuntary. Particularly after litigation has actually begun, the witness may be compelled to appear and testify pursuant to subpoena. In most instances, this would be a subpoena *ad testificandum*, meaning literally "come in and give testimony." A subpoena is a written legal order directing a person to appear in court or in some other legal proceeding (e.g., a deposition) to give testimony. Subpoenas that have been properly "served" upon the witness according to court rules generally have the force of law. Failure or refusal to respond as directed subjects the person to sanctions - usually a bench warrant for physical arrest and a citation for contempt of court. The compulsory aspects of a subpoena cannot be taken lightly. When in doubt concerning the propriety of a subpoena, a person subpoenaed as a witness should immediately consult with appropriate legal counsel.

Any professional who provides a service to a client is a potential witness in a legal proceeding. Therapists are quite likely to be called as witnesses to testify - in most instances, as "expert witnesses." This suggests that the person's testimony would not necessarily be based on first-hand knowledge (direct observation of facts material to a case), but most likely would be based on the "opinion" of the witness concerning an issue material to the case.

When professionals, such as therapists, are subpoenaed to testify in a legal proceeding, they probably will receive a subpoena *duces tecum*, which literally means "come in and bring your records." Implicit in the subpoena is also the command to "come in and testify." Like its counterpart, the subpoena *ad testificandum*, the subpoena *duces tecum* has the full force of law and is subject to sanctions if the subpoenaed witness fails or refuses to honor its terms.

Professionals, such as therapists, should concern themselves not only with the legal sufficiency of service of the commanding document, the subpoena, but also with such matters as (a) which party to the proceeding is issuing the command; (b) whether the information sought by the subpoenaing party is privileged against disclosure without express permission of the client; (c) whether the documents sought have been identified with reasonable certainty; and (d) whether the documents sought are in actual existence in the hands of the subpoenaed party at the time the subpoena is served.

In any event, a therapist who is subpoenaed *ad testificandum* or *duces tecum* should seek advice from a responsible legal advisor (this may even be the lawyer issuing the subpoena if there is no conflict of interest between them) before responding. Unless there is a specific agreement or understanding concerning response to a subpoena, the subpoenaed witness is clearly obligated to appear at the time and place specified and to produce the documents called for in a subpoena *duces tecum.*

Therapists, as professionals, are generally compensated at a specific contract rate. When subpoenaed as professional or expert witnesses, they are entitled to compensation at their established or contract rate - in contrast with ordinary witnesses, who are compensated only at the statutory witness rate (usually a nominal sum, which in most jurisdictions averages between $10 and $20 a day). In some instances, specific court authorization must be given to pay expert witness fees. However, the therapist as expert witness is entitled to appropriate compensation and should make it clear to the subpoenaing party that professional services require it. This compensation would include specific charges for file review, client interviews, telephone calls, correspondence, report preparation, travel, and maintenance expense incidental to the testimony in depositions and at trials. It is quite appropriate for the therapist, as an expert witness, to require prepayment of charges for services incidental to the therapist's testimony in any legal proceeding. There are times, however, when the compulsory aspects of a subpoena would require court intervention on the issue of prepayment. This is something that normally would be handled by lawyers representing one or the other parties to a legal proceeding.

It should be made clear that any payment received by a therapist for fees and costs as an expert witness is not payment for the opinion or conclusion given by the witness. The opinion of a professional should not be "for sale." Fees and costs must relate legitimately to identifiable professional services and incidental expenses for appearance as a witness.

On the surface, most subpoenas will require a witness to report to a deposition or a court proceeding at the beginning session. In theory, this could result in a witness' remaining in attendance for unnecessary hours, days, or even weeks. For the professional whose time is money, such uncontrolled scheduling can mean a waste of time, unnecessary interruption of the professional's usual schedule, and greater costs to the party subpoenaing the professional as a witness.

A deposition is a formal proceeding in pretrial "discovery" that permits the lawyers to subpoena and question witnesses under oath with a court reporter present, but without a judicial officer presiding. The verbatim record is usually transcribed and filed with the court and may be used as evidence to impeach a witness by "prior inconsistent recorded testimony." Court rules in most jurisdictions permit a deposition witness the privilege of reviewing a transcript of that witness' testimony and filing an addendum with corrections of transcription errors or of "misspoken" words before signing the transcript. Most court reporters will ask whether a witness "waives signature" on the transcript. A witness may decline the privilege of reviewing a transcript before it is filed. As a general rule, qualified court reporters are highly professional. They transcribe and report accurately. Many lawyers and witnesses will "waive signature" when they have no reason to review the transcript.

Therapists as witnesses are cautioned against routinely waiving signatures on depositions. They should, in most instances, review the verbatim transcript for accuracy and also obtain a copy of the document for their files and refreshment of recollection.

Formal court proceedings, of course, are generally understood by most persons. This is the proceeding in which a judicial officer (usually a judge, referee, hearing officer, or commissioner) presides. In most instances, there are a clerk and a court reporter. If it is a jury case, there is a jury. The proceedings generally are conducted according to the "rules of evidence." Until recently, dramatic portrayals of court proceedings in motion pictures and television have been notoriously inept and misleading. One program that comes close to dramatically portraying the real world of the courtroom is the National Broadcasting Company's television series "L. A. Law." Judges, lawyers, jurors, witnesses, and issues are treated with intelligence and realism. In its present posture, it can be recommended as a positive example of the legal process.

As a matter of courtesy, most lawyers are willing to agree that a professional appearing as a witness can be scheduled for a particular hour and date. In fact, it is not uncommon for judges in court proceedings to announce that the proceedings are being interrupted so that a witness may be called out of turn to facilitate his or her professional schedule.

Subpoena *duces tecum* generally by their wording requires that records to be produced must be original records. This is another area that readily lends itself to courtesy negotiation. Where records are maintained on

170

hard copy, it is fairly simple to offer clear and exact photocopies of original documents with the understanding that the originals will be available for inspection and comparison, if necessary. Most jurisdictions have statutes that permit photocopies of documents to be admitted in place of originals if the accuracy of the reproduction can be reasonably verified. This can usually be established by the testimony of the person presenting the documents to the effect that the person has compared the photocopies with the originals and that they are identical. Modern photocopying processes permit this to be done with confidence, although the person receiving photocopies of documents should remain vigilant to (and at times be quite suspicious of) the possibility of alteration between an original document and the photocopied document by the use of "white-out" or photoblocking tape. Any person offering photocopies as substitutes for originals should be honor bound in asserting that the photocopies are accurate representations of the originals. While the assertion may initially be informal, it would be made under oath when the person is testifying in a deposition or in a court proceeding.

With the exception of government investigations such as grand jury proceedings, there is generally no legal compulsion available to require a person to give evidence or testify as a witness prior to the actual filing of a lawsuit. Government investigations are not within the scope of this discussion.

Once a lawsuit is filed, however, the lawyers for either party in most jurisdictions generally have the authority to issue subpoenas, which must be honored by the person subpoenaed. Failure or refusal to honor a subpoena properly served subjects the recipient to severe sanctions. Many lawyers still include the somewhat archaic language in subpoenas directing the person to appear and "fail not at your peril."

One of the first things anyone should do upon learning that that person will be a witness in a legal proceeding is to find out what the case is about. Cases are formally initiated by "pleading," most commonly in the nature of (a) a summons and complaint filed by the plaintiff against a defendant, and (b) an answer filed by the defendant. There are at times, of course, cross-complaints and counterclaims, but the parties generally remain the same. The complaint and answer at least provide information concerning the parties to the proceeding, the general facts underlying the case, the claims made by the plaintiff, and the answer, or defense, given by the defendants. The names of the lawyers representing each party are prominently identified on the pleadings by court rule.

A therapist generally would be called to testify in a legal proceeding in connection with professional services rendered to a specific patient. It thus is essential for the therapist to know which party is calling the professional as a witness and the identity of the patient. Unless the therapist is being called as a witness by the patient, serious questions of confidentiality and privilege immediately arise. Even if called by the patient, the therapist should obtain in writing some form of waiver for necessary disclosure of confidential information in the course of the proceeding.

At times a therapist may be called upon to conduct an interview and prepare a report on a person who has not previously been a patient. This is generally done for a specific purpose in connection with a particular issue in a legal proceeding.

A therapist also may be called upon to evaluate reports prepared by other professionals without necessarily interviewing the subject of the report. This is usually done when an opinion on an abstract issue is sought from the professional.

Legal proceedings may involve depositions in the course of pretrial discovery or actual trials in court. Trials may be before judges without a jury or before a jury. The basic rules of procedure are essentially the same, particularly with reference to the order of presentation of evidence.

As a general rule, the initiating party in a lawsuit (usually referred to as the Plaintiff or Petitioner) is the first in order and the responding party (usually referred to as Defendant or Respondent) is the second in order. The following represents a typical process in trial.

1. Pretrial conference with lawyers and judge.
2. Jury selection in a jury trial.
3. Opening statement by plaintiff (a general outline of what the plaintiff expects its evidence to show).
4. Opening statement by defendant (a general outline of what the defendant expects its evidence to show).

5. Presentation of plaintiff's case: examination of plaintiff's witnesses by plaintiff (called "direct examination") followed by examination of each witness by defendant (called "cross-examination"). "Redirect examination" and "recross-examination" sometimes take place.

6. Challenge by the defendant to the sufficiency of evidence presented by the plaintiff. If the challenge is granted, the case is dismissed. In most instances, however, the challenge is denied and the case proceeds.

7. Presentation of defendant's case: examination of defendant's witnesses by defendant (called "direct examination") followed by examination of each witness by plaintiff (called "cross-examination"). "Redirect examination" and "recross-examination" sometimes take place.

8. Sometimes the plaintiff will present "rebuttal testimony." The process of examination and cross-examination is the same as in the plaintiff's case referred to in Item 5.

9. In a jury trial, written instructions (agreed upon by the lawyers and the judge) are read to the jury by the judge. This step would not occur where the case is tried to a judge without a jury.

10. Closing argument by plaintiff (an editorial argument summarizing the evidence presented and applying applicable law to the facts).

11. Closing argument by defendant (an editorial argument summarizing the evidence presented and applying applicable law to the facts).

12. Rebuttal argument by plaintiff (direct rebuttal to closing argument of defendant).

13. Jury retires to deliberate in jury cases.

14. In trials before a judge without a jury, the judge may then make a decision in the case.

15. In jury cases, the jury, after deliberation, will return to court with a verdict. The verdict of the jury is then formally announced in open court.

Lawyers are required by the rules of professional conduct (the lawyers' code of professional responsibility) to be courteous to all participants in court proceedings. At times, however, firmness and aggressive pursuit of a client's case by a lawyer may be interpreted as discourtesy. Vigorous cross-examination is not in itself discourteous. However, discourtesy sometimes is masked as "vigorous cross-examination." Serious matters of discourtesy should not arise. Witnesses are entitled to be treated with respect. If a lawyer fails to do so, the matter should be reported through an appropriate process.

THE FEDERAL RULES OF EVIDENCE

For many years, court proceedings were governed by an amorphous conglomeration of English common-law principles, statutes (including the Napoleonic Code, which applies in Louisiana), local court rules, and provincial practice. The order of presentation of evidence was essentially uniform. The rules of evidence, however, would vary from jurisdiction to jurisdiction, from court to court, and from courtroom to courtroom.

Lawyers and judges of an earlier generation were accustomed to the rules of evidence most popularly articulated by Dean John Henry Wigmore of Harvard Law School first published in 1904, whose treatise was the "bible" of evidence until the 1970s. The states of Oregon, California, and Georgia had earlier adopted statutory codes of evidence. Louisiana has always followed the Napoleonic Code.

The American Law Institute Model Code of Evidence followed in 1939, but was not adopted in any state. Then came the National Conference of Commissioners on Uniform State Laws, which adopted the *Uniform Rules of Evidence* in 1953. By 1968, the Uniform Rules had been adopted only in Kansas and New Jersey. Utah adopted them in 1971. California adopted its own evidence rules in 1967.

In 1965, Chief Justice Earl Warren of the U.S. Supreme Court appointed an advisory committee to study and make recommendations concerning the *Preliminary Report of the Special Committee on Evidence* published in February 1962, which, after comments from lawyers and judges, concluded that federal evidence rules were feasible and desirable. The advisory committee's preliminary draft of the *Federal Rules of Evidence* was published in 1969 and forwarded to the Supreme Court.

After a fairly complicated process of review, comments, and evaluations, the *Federal Rules of Evidence* were approved by the Supreme Court and by Congress, effective July 1, 1975. The National Conference of Commissioners on Uniform State Laws adopted a new version of

174

the *Uniform Rules of Evidence* patterned on the Congressional (House) version of the Federal Rules in 1974, adopting the numbering and language of the Federal Rules.

The *Federal Rules of Evidence* inspired adoption of similar or identical rules in many state jurisdictions. A 1983 tabulation of states substantially adopting the *Federal Rules of Evidence* includes Alaska, Arizona, Arkansas, Colorado, Delaware, Florida, Hawaii, Maine, Michigan, Minnesota, Montana, Nebraska, Nevada, New Mexico, North Dakota, Ohio, Oklahoma, Oregon, South Dakota, Texas, Vermont, Washington, Wisconsin, and Wyoming. Puerto Rico and the armed services have adopted versions of the *Federal Rules.* As a practical matter, then, the *Federal Rules of Evidence* provide a fairly reliable basis for determining the rules of evidence that will apply in most jurisdictions.

The *Federal Rules of Evidence* (28 United States Code, Sections 101 through 1103) provide a general outline for the conduct of trials that may be of some benefit to the nonlawyer witness who is not familiar with court procedures. The following rules seem to be of particular relevance.

Rule 611. **Mode and Order of Interrogation and Presentation.**

(a) *Control by Court.* The court shall exercise reasonable control over the mode and order of interrogating witnesses and presenting evidence so as to (1) make the interrogation and presentation effective for the ascertainment of the truth, (2) avoid needless consumption of time, and (3) protect witnesses from harassment or undue embarrassment.

(b) *Scope of Cross-Examination.* Cross-examination should be limited to the subject matter of the direct examination and matters affecting the credibility of the witness. The court may, in the exercise of discretion, permit inquiry into additional matters as if on direct examination.

(c) *Leading Questions.* Leading questions should not be used on the direct examination of a witness except as may be necessary to develop his testimony. Ordinarily leading questions should be permitted on cross-examination. When a party calls a hostile witness, an adverse party, or a witness identified with an adverse party, interrogation may be by leading questions.

Rule 612. **Writing Used to Refresh Memory**.

Except as otherwise provided in criminal proceedings by Section 3500 of title 18, United States Code, if a witness uses a writing to refresh his memory for the purpose of testifying, either--

(1) while testifying, or
(2) before testifying, if the court in its discretion determines it is necessary in the interests of justice,

an adverse party is entitled to have the writing produced at the hearing, to inspect it, to cross-examine the witness thereon, and to introduce in evidence those portions which relate to the testimony of the witness. If it is claimed that the writing contains matters not related to the subject matter of the testimony, the court shall examine the writing *in camera*, excise any portions not so related, and order delivery of the remainder to the party entitled thereto. Any portion withheld over objections shall be preserved and made available to the appellate court in the event of an appeal. If a writing is not produced or delivered pursuant to order under this rule, the court shall make any order justice requires, except that in criminal cases when the prosecution elects not to comply, the order shall be one striking the testimony or, if the court in its discretion determines that the interests of justice so require, declaring a mistrial.

Rule 613. **Prior Statements of Witnesses**.

(a) *Examining Witness Concerning Prior Statements*. In examining a witness concerning a prior statement made by him, whether written or not, the statement need not be shown nor its contents disclosed to him at that time, but on request the same shall be shown or disclosed to opposing counsel.
(b) *Extrinsic Evidence of Prior Inconsistent Statement of Witness*. Extrinsic evidence of a prior

inconsistent statement by a witness is not admissible unless the witness is afforded an opportunity to explain or deny the same and the opposite party is afforded an opportunity to interrogate him thereon, or the interests of justice otherwise require . . . .

Rule 614. **Calling and Interrogation of Witnesses by Court.**

(a) *Calling by Court.* The court may, on its own motion or at the suggestion of a party, call witnesses, and all parties are entitled to cross-examine witnesses thus called.

(b) *Interrogation by Court.* The court may interrogate witnesses, whether called by itself or by a party.

(c) *Objections.* Objections to the calling of witnesses by the court or to interrogation by it may be made at the time or at the next available opportunity when the jury is not present.

Rule 615. **Exclusion of Witnesses.**

At the request of a party the court shall order witnesses excluded so that they cannot hear the testimony of other witnesses, and it may make the order of its own motion. This rule does not authorize exclusion of (1) a party who is a natural person, or (2) an officer or employee of a party which is not a natural person designated as its representative by its attorney, or (3) a person whose presence is shown by a party to be essential to the presentation of his cause.

One area of evidence law that is of particular significance to therapists but is not included in the *Federal Rules of Evidence* is that of *privilege*, that is, the privilege against disclosure of confidential communications. Deleted from the preliminary draft of the *Federal Rules of Evidence* was Proposed Rule 504 entitled "Psychotherapist-Patient Privilege." In the final version of the rules, this area was left to state law, common-law rules, and more general principles of evidence.

It is worthwhile, however, to recite Proposed Federal Rule of Evidence 504 for guidance purposes only inasmuch as it is still a fair representation of principles relating to confidential communications between psychotherapists and patients. It must be remembered that this rule was *not* adopted.

Proposed Rule 504 [Not Adopted]. **Psychotherapist-Patient Privilege.**

(a) *Definitions.*

(1) A "patient" is a person who consults or is examined or interviewed by a psychotherapist.

(2) A "psychotherapist" is (A) a person authorized to practice medicine in any state or nation, or reasonably believed by the patient so to be, while engaged in the diagnosis or treatment of a mental or emotional condition, including drug addiction, or (B) a person licensed or certified as a psychologist under the laws of any state or nation, while similarly engaged.

(3) A communication is "confidential" if not intended to be disclosed to third persons other than those present to further the interest of the patient in the consultation, examination, or interview, or persons reasonably necessary for the transmission of the communication, or persons who are participating in the diagnosis and treatment under the direction of the psychotherapist, including members of the patient's family.

(b) *General rule of Privilege.*

A patient has a privilege to refuse to disclose and to prevent any other person from disclosing confidential communications, made for the purpose of diagnosis or treatment of his mental or emotional condition, including drug addiction, among himself, his psychotherapist, or persons who are participating in the diagnosis or treatment under the direction of the psychotherapist, including members of the patient's family.

(c) *Who may claim the privilege.*

The privilege may be claimed by the patient, by his guardian or conservator, or by the personal representative of a deceased patient. The person who was the psychotherapist may claim the privilege but only on behalf of the patient. His authority so to do is presumed in the absence of evidence to the contrary.

(d) *Exceptions.*

(1) *Proceedings for hospitalization.* There is no privilege under this rule for communications relevant to an issue in proceedings to hospitalize the patient for mental illness, if the psychotherapist in the course of diagnosis or treatment has determined that the patient is in need of hospitalization.

(2) *Examination by order of judge.* If the judge orders an examination of the mental or emotional condition of the patient, communications made in the course thereof are not privileged under this rule with respect to the particular purpose for which the examination is ordered unless the judge orders otherwise.

(3) *Condition an element of claim or defense.* There is no privilege under this rule as to communications relevant to an issue of the mental or emotional condition of the patient in any proceeding in which he relies upon the condition as an element of his claim or defense, or, after the patient's death, in any proceeding in which any party relies upon the condition as an element of his claim or defense.

A therapist anticipating testimony in any legal proceeding should consult with appropriate legal counsel to clarify the law relating to privileged communications in a particular jurisdiction. The therapist should also clearly determine whether the lawyer subpoenaing represents the therapist's client or the adversary party.

It is important to call attention to the difference between the *personal privilege*, which is used to exclude evidence, and the *exclusionary rules*, which are also used to exclude evidence. Evidence excluded because of *personal privilege* is not excluded because of a danger that the testimony will be untrustworthy or that the trier of fact will be incapable of evaluating it. In fact, the chances are that evidence excluded under a valid claim of a personal privilege probably would be admissible under the rules of evidence.

When a privilege exists, an individual may not be compelled to disclose information about a particular event. This is somewhat inconsistent with the noble search for truth that is the hallmark of our judicial system. As with the Fifth Amendment privilege against self-incrimination (a commonly understood personal privilege), a privilege generally brings into focus a value considered of more significance than the mere search for truth. Professor David W. Louisell in a 1956 *Tulane Law Review* article summarized Dean Wigmore's comment on the balance fostered by this inconsistency:

1. The communications must originate in a *confidence* that they will not be disclosed;
2. This element of *confidentiality must be essential* to the full and satisfactory maintenance of the relation between the parties;
3. The *relation* must be one which in the opinion of the community ought to be sedulously fostered; and
4. The *injury* that would inure to the relation by the disclosure of the communications must be *greater than the benefit* thereby gained for the correct disposal of litigation.

In general, the courts tend to disfavor most privileges unless they are clearly articulated by statute or rule. It seems that the world is concretely divided between those who favor privileges and those who do not favor privileges.

According to Carlson, Imwinkelried, and Kionka (*Materials for the Study of Evidence*, 1983), in certain types of proceedings the holder has certain privileges with respect to certain types of information unless (a) the holder has waived the privilege or (b) there is a special exception to the privilege's scope. They reduce all privilege issues to these six questions.

1. *To what type of proceedings does the privilege apply?*

The courts usually say that the rationale for creating privileges is that privileges encourage full and free communication between persons standing in certain special relationships (such as husband-wife, priest-penitent, physician-patient, attorney-client, and psychotherapist-patient). The courts assume that it would affect that freedom of communication if privileges did not exist. The practical questions that arise are: Would the persons standing in those special relationships communicate less freely if there were no privilege? To what extent? Is the supposed decrease in the flow of information great enough to justify the obstructive effect the privileges have on the search for truth?

2. *Who is the holder of the privilege?*

If legally irrelevant evidence or incompetent opinion is offered at a trial, the opposing party automatically has a right to object. The opposing party, however, does not have the same automatic right to object on the grounds of privilege. A party to a proceeding is not necessarily the holder of a privilege and the holder of a privilege is not necessarily a party. However, a party may be the holder of a privilege and the holder of a privilege may be a party. Confusing? Yes.

A party who holds a privilege and who is not a party to a lawsuit may intervene for purposes of asserting the privilege if the testimony sought would violate a privilege existing between the holder and the party testifying. In the case of most professional privileges, the person seeking the service is the holder. Professionals believing that information sought from them in testimony is privileged have an obligation at least to call it to the attention of the judicial officer, who probably will respect an assertion in good faith and will allow the privilege even though it does not belong to the professional asserting it.

3. *What is the nature of the privilege?*

The various privileges include three different rights: (a) the right personally to refuse to disclose the privileged information; (b) the right to prevent a third party from making an unauthorized disclosure of the privileged communication; and (c) the right to prevent trial comment on the invocation of the privilege.

4. *What type of information is privileged?*

There must first be a *communication*. The policy underlying the creation of privileges is the promotion of communication between persons standing in certain relationships. The communication must be *confidential*. As a general rule, the courts will look to see whether at the time of the communication that parties had physical privacy and intended the communication to be confidential.

If the communicating parties did not manifest an intention to maintain secrecy at the time of communication, the courts will not confer confidentiality later in the courtroom. If an eavesdropper overhears a confidential communication, the privilege is usually vitiated and the eavesdropper may testify concerning it.

The party claiming the privilege must show that at the time of communication there was an intent to maintain secrecy in the future. The communication must be a confidential communication between the parties. It must be a communication that occurs between properly related parties and is "incidental to the relationship."

5. *Has there been a waiver of the privilege?*

A determination of privilege is not absolute. A party opposing the claim can defeat the privilege by showing either a waiver or a special exception. The courts will generally find a waiver where the holder discloses a substantial part of the privileged information. Normally a waiver must be free and voluntary. However, some courts will treat inadvertent disclosure as a waiver and other courts require a stronger intent to waive.

6. *Is there any pertinent special exception?*

In answering this, we must consider (a) the interpretative intent of the holder, (b) fairness, and (c) countervailing social policy.

As a practical matter, most psychiatrists and psychologists who testify as expert witnesses in legal proceedings would be testifying concerning communications with a patient. This immediately suggests a confidential communications privilege - probably by statute. Almost all jurisdictions have specific statutory physician-patient communications privileges. Some have specific psychotherapist-patient communications privileges, and some have specific psychologist-patient communications privileges. Resolution of the privileged communications issue should be one of the early concerns of any therapist who expects to be subpoenaed as a witness.

The *Federal Rules of Evidence* are more important for what they do contain than for what they do not contain. A general familiarity with pertinent rules will help the nonlawyer witness to function better in the legal environment. The following *Federal Rules of Evidence* are particularly significant.

Rule 701. Opinion Testimony By Lay Witnesses.

If the witness is not testifying as an expert, his testimony in the form of opinions or inferences is limited to those opinions or inferences which are (a) rationally based on the perception of the witness and (b) helpful to a clear understanding of his testimony or the determination of a fact in issue.

Rule 702. Testimony by Experts.

If scientific, technical, or other specialized knowledge will assist the trier of fact to understand the evidence or to determine a fact in issue, a witness qualified as an expert by knowledge, skill, experience, training, or education, may testify thereto in the form of an opinion or otherwise.

Rule 703. Bases of Opinion Testimony By Experts.

The facts or data in the particular case upon which an expert bases an opinion or inference may be those perceived by or made known to him at or before the hearing. If of a type reasonably relied upon by experts in the particular field in forming opinions or inferences upon the subject, the facts or data need not be admissible in evidence.

Rule 705. **Disclosure of Facts or Data Underlying Expert Opinion.**

The expert may testify in terms of opinion or inference and give his reasons therefor without prior disclosure of the underlying facts or data, unless the court requires otherwise. The expert may in any event be required to disclose the underlying facts or data on cross-examination.

Rule 104. **Preliminary Questions.**

(a) *Questions of Admissibility Generally.* Preliminary questions concerning the qualification of a person to be a witness, the existence of a privilege, or the admissibility of evidence shall be determined by the court, subject to the provisions of subdivision (b). In making its determination it is not bound by the rules of evidence except those with respect to privileges.

(b) *Relevancy Conditioned on Fact.* When the relevancy of evidence depends upon the fulfillment of a condition of fact, the court shall admit it upon, or subject to, the introduction of evidence sufficient to support a finding of the fulfillment of the condition.

. . . .

One way expert testimony is presented is to have the expert testify about facts of personal knowledge, such as objective observations by an examining physician or observation by a psychologist of the behavior of a patient during an interview. More often there is no opportunity for personal knowledge or observation by the expert witness. In that event, the expert must rely on data or opinions gathered by others.

Some courts in common-law jurisdictions do not allow experts to rely on data gathered by others, however. Others do, but instruct the jury that such testimony is not to be considered for its truth. The *Federal Rules of Evidence* (see Rule 703) provide that an expert witness must rely on data that are not otherwise admissible in evidence. The important thing is that the data are the type reasonably relied upon by experts in the particular field, such as a learned treatise or a learned article written by an acknowledged expert on the subject. Under Federal Rule of Evidence 803 (18), a learned treatise is admissible as an exception to the hearsay rule:

> The following are not excluded by the hearsay rule, even though the declarant is available as a witness:
>
> . . . .
>
> (18) *Learned treatises.* To the extent called to the attention of an expert witness upon cross-examination or relied upon by him in direct examination, statements contained in published treatises, periodicals, or pamphlets on a subject of history, medicine, or other science or art, established as a reliable authority by the testimony or admission of the witness or by other expert testimony or by judicial notice. If admitted, the statements may be read into evidence but may not be received as exhibits.
>
> . . . .

An expert witness may be asked to state an opinion by assuming the existence of stated facts, all of which must be the subject of other proof, or by assuming the facts testified to by other witnesses (the expert would have either been in court and heard the testimony or have been provided an opportunity to review a verbatim transcript). When relying on the testimony of other witnesses, it is important that the facts not be controverted so that the trier of fact may rely upon the circumstance that what the expert is assuming as a basis for expert opinion is indeed true.

An expert witness may be asked a hypothetical question as the basis for an expert opinion. The basis would be clear from the question itself. A hypothetical question is one that asks the witness to assume certain facts (based upon a summary of evidence in the record or, at the least, a summary of some evidence in the record and some evidence not in the record that subsequently is to be connected by evidence) as a basis upon which to give an opinion. Hypothetical questions should be carefully reasoned out, written out, and structured so that they do not unintentionally omit relevant facts or include facts not of record. Unfortunately, not all lawyers understand this. All too frequently, they try to create a hypothetical question as they are asking it. The expert witness should be wary of that type of question.

An expert witness may be asked to given an opinion based on personal knowledge (such as examining something or observing something or drawing on the witness' reservoir of knowledge about a particular subject). In jurisdictions that follow a strict rule on expert testimony based on personal knowledge, if it develops on cross-examination that the witness really did not have the requisite personal knowledge, the testimony is subject to being stricken because the foundation that permits the testimony has been removed.

The word "foundation" in the presentation of evidence is not altogether different from the dictionary definition of the word: "that on which something is founded" or "the basis or ground of anything" or "the natural or pre-pared ground or base on which some structure rests" (*Webster's New World Dictionary*, 1960). In a legal proceeding, the word "foundation" means the admissible evidence necessary to move from point A to point B in the orderly presentation of evidence under the rules. A common form of objection from opposing counsel would be stated: "Objection - no foundation" or "Objection - improper foundation."

The foundation for the testimony of an expert witness requires evidence concerning the identity of the witness; the education, training, and experience of the witness, including membership in learned societies; and the witness' background in the field that is the subject of expert testimony. On occasion, opposing counsel may wish to question the witness on *voir dire* (ask preliminary questions out of turn) to explore further the witness' qualifications or lack of qualifications. Although a layperson may give an opinion under the rules of evidence, this opinion is to be distinguished from that of an expert, who must meet the foundation requirements to qualify as such.

A rather practical article entitled "Psychiatrists and Psychologists: Using Expert Witnesses" and written by Seattle trial attorney J. A. George was published in the *Seattle-King County Bar Bulletin* in October 1982. The following excerpts from George's article seem to have some relevance to therapists who may be called to testify as witnesses in legal proceedings:

186

Preparing the Witness

Witness preparation should begin when the expert is first retained or notified of the appointment. The objective of the evaluation and the legal requirements should be discussed. Continuing contact with an expert is suggested if the evaluation is ongoing.

In most instances, a written report is advisable. Following receipt, the report should be discussed with the expert. A second opinion may be appropriate. If no written report is supplied, the expert should be deposed. As a general rule, depositions of all expert witnesses should be taken. There are two schools of thought regarding the extent to which an expert's position should be challenged in deposition. The general rule is to expose weaknesses and thus challenge the expert outside of the presence of jury or judge. At the same time, it removes the element of surprise and gives the expert an opportunity to cover the weaknesses and prepare for cross-examination. The best result is to discover the weaknesses without warning the adversary.

Prior to examination, the expert should be well prepared. An outline of specifically phrased questions for direct examination should be provided. The expert should also have an advance opportunity to suggest questions and respond to the phraseology of questions needed to elicit information supporting the opinion or recommendations.

Even if the expert has testified previously, it may be useful to review the trial process and to describe the courtroom style of opposing counsel. If the expert has never or seldom testified, the above topics should be discussed in great depth, especially the latter. Many experts appreciate the opportunity to practice cross examination. The same challenges outlined below apply to expert witnesses called on direct examination.

It is also imperative to discuss what the attorney perceives as weaknesses in the opinions or recommendations and the types of questions that the opposing counsel may ask. When two or more experts will be called to testify, the expert testifying on your behalf should be shown all reports, evaluations and deposition transcripts for review and discussion.

Direct Examination

It is important for the court or jury to understand the expert's education, qualifications, specializations, type of practice, publications, university affiliations, previous testimony experience, and preferably how many times they have testified in court on both sides of similar cases. An attorney should not merely stipulate to his own expert's qualifications, especially in areas most relevant to the case at hand. A vitae for the individual ought to be offered for review by the trier of fact.

Cross-Examination

Most trial lawyers admit that cross-examination is their greatest weakness and especially the cross-examination of expert witnesses. Lifted from every expert trial lawyer who has ever given a seminar, cut a tape, or written a book, are the following general rules:

Know when not to cross-examine: Even though some witnesses should be excused after direct examination with a simple statement "No questions, your Honor," almost without exception, expert witnesses must be cross-examined. This is the rule, even if the only purpose of cross examination is to raise doubt as to the reality or validity of psychiatric or psychological evaluations.

Know when to stop cross-examinations: All trial lawyers will sometime ask a question that provides a lead in for the expert to justify or explain away previous problems or weakness brought out in cross examination.

Never ask questions to which you do not know the answer: As outlined above, the depositions of expert witnesses should be taken so that answers to questions posed in court are anticipated. To acquire such knowledge is one of the main purposes for deposing the expert witness before trial. Avoiding unanticipated answers is especially critical in front of a jury where much information may come into evidence before the examiner can prevent the answer. "Unringing the bell" through judicial rulings to disregard information is not a good method of eliminating damaging information.

Never give open ended questions to an expert witness: Expert witnesses can be most harmful to an attorney's case and particularly those in psychology and psychiatry. If a psychiatrist is asked "why?" on cross examination, every piece of information that was kept out in direct examination through objections will be volunteered. This allows the expert to speculate and again to explain away any concerns the jurors or judge may have.

Exclude expert witnesses from the courtroom: It is beneficial to exclude all witnesses from the courtroom, since it precludes comparison and reaffirmation of testimony. It keeps the expert from observing and listening to another expert testimony and anticipating or modifying weaknesses in his own evaluation and presentation.

The objective of cross-examination is to discredit testimony of the opposing expert witness. Despite the availability of many reference books, the average lawyer will rarely be able to acquire sufficient information to effectively discredit an expert's academic knowledge. The best approach to cross-examining psychiatric and psychological experts is to challenge the field of psychiatry itself. The fields of psychiatry and psychology are still in their infancy and devoid of validated scientific base. Experts renowned in the same field will publish theories diametrically opposed. The definitions and diagnoses of illness in *The American Psychiatric Association Diagnostic and Statistical Manual of Mental Disorders* are determined by a majority vote by the American Psychiatric Association. Studies have shown that experts evaluating the exact same case may agree on assessment and diagnosis no more than forty-five to sixty percent of the time.

When cross-examining an expert on theory, the diligent attorney can quickly elicit its speculative and uncertain character. Most experts are willing to agree that the field lacks scientific foundation and even consensus on key questions. To challenge the theoretical, it must first be ascertained through deposition as outlined above. Once determined, it can almost always be attacked . . . .

These same challenges may be directed toward the psychologist who attempts to verify opinions through psychological testing. These tests supply slightly more objective data, but are still challengeable. There are seven to nine tests that can be included in the battery of testing and the examiner should have some knowledge of them. The scoring of these tests is considered to be scientific, yet psychologists disagree as to the requisite lower limit of reliability. There are extensive scientific theoretical challenges that can be made, depending upon the particular facts and theories at hand.

In addition to theoretical challenges, it is possible to challenge the expert's credibility by inquiring into procedures or tests *not* conducted or people *not* interviewed. For example, in criminal cases, proximity to the time of the crime is important, since the test for legal insanity applies primarily to mental status at the time of the crime.

. . . .

Both juries and judges have often relied totally upon psychiatric and psychological experts to render decisions significantly affecting the lives of individuals and families. This article hopefully points out the need for lawyers to require the expert witness to discuss the lack of scientific foundation and verification for their opinions as part of the evaluation.

Since psychiatric and psychological experts provide the least scientific information of any experts usually called to testify, they are challengeable by questioning lack of theory or by examining problems specific to each individual case . . . . Even though these challenges may be more effective before juries than judges, most judges will admit that although the expert testimony weighs heavily in their decision, it is only one aspect to be considered. Just as juries have ignored psychiatric testimony, judges can decide not to follow the recommendations presented by an expert.*

It may provide some comfort to nonlawyer professional witnesses to learn that lawyers can be just as intimidated by professional expert witnesses as the witnesses can be intimidated by lawyers. There is actually no real basis for this intimidation if each person has a fair understanding of the processes followed by the other in performing that person's function.

Lawyers need to become more knowledgeable about the technical aspects of psychological and psychiatric matters such as post-traumatic stress disorder, a relatively new term in the legal and behavioral science fields. In addition to more cooperative education between the discipline of law and those of the behavioral sciences, psychiatrists and psychologists can help to educate lawyers.

An article in the March 1988 issue of *Trial*, published by the Association of Trial Lawyers of America, is a case in point. The article, "Post-Traumatic Stress Disorder: The Unrecognized Syndrome," written by Ari Kiev, MD, a New York City psychiatrist and clinical professor of psychiatry at Cornell University Medical College specializing in forensic psychiatry, describes characteristics of the post-traumatic stress disorder to alert lawyers to ask questions that will elicit details to support their clients' cases.

ADVICE FOR THE THERAPIST AS WITNESS

The confident therapist who is fully prepared and knowledgeable about the area of expertise involved in the testimony need not fear the onslaught of legal inquiry. The reality is that the therapist as an expert witness should be infinitely more knowledgeable about the subject than any practicing lawyer. Although the process of inquiry in legal proceedings is something of a game, there are well-defined rules that are designed to assure that the search for truth follows an orderly process. The lawyers, who are the principal performers in the litigation game, are refereed by a judicial officer (usually a judge) and

---

*Note. From "Psychiatrists and Psychologists: Using Expert Witnesses" by J. A. George, 1982, October, Seattle-King County Bar Bulletin, pp. 1, 13. Reprinted by permission.

are required to question witnesses on direct examination and cross-examination in a fair manner and with the courtesy required in a courtroom.

The therapist who will testify as an expert witness need have no real apprehension about the testimonial experience if the therapist is reasonably familiar with court proceedings and the nature of the case, and is absolutely familiar with the subject matter of the therapist's expertise.

There may be times when a therapist who has been subpoenaed, or expects to be subpoenaed, to testify in a proceeding may wish to consult that person's own lawyer concerning the therapist's legal rights and obligations. Utilizing that resource, if available, is highly recommended when there are any uncertainties about the process.

What can the expert witness expect from a jury? Lawsuits are tried either before a jury with a judge presiding, or before a judge (or other judicial officer) without a jury. Most juries consist of 12 persons, although the rules in some jurisdictions permit juries with fewer members. Where there is a jury, the jury is the "trier of fact." It is the responsibility of the jury to listen to the evidence presented through testimony and documents, listen to instructions on the law given by the judge, deliberate on the facts and the law, and then make a decision. The judge will give the specific instructions as to how to do this.

Jury instructions remind the jurors that they are the finders of fact in the search for truth. They may also be instructed to consider such things as the education, training, experience, knowledge, and sources of information provided by expert witnesses. Jurors are not provided with any magic device by which they reach their conclusions. Presumably, they need only be alert and intelligent, and have the capacity to observe what occurs in the courtroom.

Jurors tend to watch witnesses carefully. They will observe a witness' appearance (grooming, choice of clothing, and choice of colors) and body language (posture, eye contact, and facial expressions), and heed witness' facility of language (clearness, conciseness, articulation, and directness). They also will note the witness' response to the lawyers questioning them ("friendly" lawyer on direct examination and "antagonistic" lawyer on cross-examination), as well as the witness' confidence in assertions made in response to questions (the witness appears knowledgeable, informed, and understanding of the subject matter).

The qualified expert witness who is knowledgeable about the subject matter, is fully prepared to give testimony in a case, answers questions with self-assurance, and conveys a sense of sincerity and intelligence while testifying need have no fear of the experience of testifying in court before a jury. In the final analysis, jurors expect expert witnesses to be sincere and well-informed, able to communicate in language laypersons can understand, and courteous to both friendly and antagonistic lawyers who question them in the course of their testimony.

Charles Z. Smith, JD, received his BS degree from Temple University and his JD degree from the University of Washington, Seattle. He was a principal in a Seattle law firm from 1983 to 1988. Since July 1988 he served as a justice of the Washington State Supreme Court. From 1973 to 1983 he was Associate Dean and Professor of Law and Director of Clinical Programs at the University of Washington School of Law. He is now Professor Emeritus of Law, a member of the Graduate Faculty, and a member of the Social Welfare Doctoral Faculty at the University of Washington. He has previously served as Judge of the Superior Court of Washington for King County, Special Assistant to the Attorney General of the United States, and Deputy Prosecuting Attorney for King County (Washington). The Honorable Charles Z. Smith may be contacted at Theodore M. Rosenblume, Charles Z. Smith, and Associates, PS, 3200 Columbia Center, 701 Fifth Avenue, Seattle, WA 98104-7097.

REFERENCES

American Bar Association. (1983). *The Litigation Manual: A Primer for Trial Lawyers* (Section of Litigation). Chicago: American Bar Association.

Broun, K. S., & Blakey, W. J. (1985). *Evidence.* St. Paul, MN: West Publishing Co.

Carlson, R. L., Imwinkelried, E. J., & Kionka, E. J. (1983). *Materials for the Study of Evidence.* Charlottesville, VA: Mitchie Co.

Federal Rules of Evidence, 28 United States Code, Sections 101 through 1103.

George, J. A. (1982, October). Psychiatrists and psychologists: Using expert witnesses. *Seattle-King County Bar Bulletin*, pp. 1, 13.

Kiev, A. (1988, March). Post-traumatic stress disorder: The unrecognized syndrome. *Trial* (Association of Trial Lawyers of America), *24*, 62-65.

Lempert, R. O., & Saltzburg, S. A. (1983). *A Modern Approach to Evidence* (2nd ed.). St. Paul, MN: West Publishing Co.

Louisell, D. W. (1956). Confidentiality, conformity and confusion: Privileges in Federal Courts today. *Tulane Law Review, 31*, 101.

McElhaney, J. W. (1981). *Trial Notebook* (Section on litigation). Chicago: American Bar Association.

Webster's New World Dictionary of the American Language (College Ed.). (1960). New York: World Publishing Co.

Appendix

Self-Evaluation of Difficulties Questionnaire

Carroll L. Meek

INSTRUCTIONS: This instrument is to be given to the patient to
take home. Encourage the person to fill it out as completely as
possible. Since some of the information may be upsetting to recall,
indicate to the patient that should it become too upsetting to
continue, that he or she should stop filling out the questionnaire
and bring it into the office to complete.

Even though the questionnaire indicates that patients can ask to
add to it as therapy/evaluation progresses, they might not do so. If
it is noticed that information which is brought up later in the evaluation has not been included on the questionnaire, ask about it.

In addition, items on the questionnaire may present the examiner
with opportunities to inquire further regarding various aspects of
the patient's life.

Post-Traumatic Stress Disorder

Please fill out the following information as <u>completely</u> as possible. It will help determine the type(s) of problems you experience. It may also help you develop ideas about things that you can do to help alleviate your difficulties.

Name_____ Date_____

Address_____ Age_____

_____ Birthdate_____

Social Security Number_____

Were you referred by someone? Yes/No (circle). If yes, who referred you?

Name_____ Title_____

Please describe, as completely as you can, the nature of your problem(s), complaint(s), and so on <u>at the present time</u>. As you describe your difficulties, please put (in parentheses after <u>each</u> problem) your age and/or the date you <u>first</u> noticed you had the problem(s):

_____

_____

_____

_____

_____

Please list problem(s) you have had <u>in the past</u> and indicate the age you were when you first noticed it/them:

	Problem	Age of Occurrence
1.	_____	_____
2.	_____	_____
3.	_____	_____
4.	_____	_____

I have/have not (circle the correct one) had therapy before <u>because</u> of this/these problem(s). If you <u>have</u> had therapy before because of your difficulties, indicate the following:

   Did it help? Yes/No (circle one). If yes, indicate what was helpful. If no, why?

   _____

   _____

   _____

   _____

198

Post-Traumatic Stress Disorder

Are you currently taking medications? Yes/No (circle one).

    If yes, what?_____

_____

    Do you take your medication as directed by a physician? Yes/No
    (circle one).

    If no, why not?_____

Have you thought of suicide before? Yes/No (circle one). If yes,
have you acted out on your suicidal impulses or thoughts? Yes/No
(circle one).

    If yes, indicate what you did and what the result was:_____

_____

_____

Please answer the following questions with a check mark in the appropriate yes/no column.

	Yes	No
1. I have trouble sleeping.............................		
a. If yes, I awaken too early......................		
b. I experience disrupted sleep (i.e., I wake up several times during the night)................		
c. I have problems falling asleep. (If yes, indicate possible reason[s])...................		

_____

_____

	Yes	No
2. I have eating problems.............................		
a. If yes, I eat too much..........................		
b. I eat too little, food does not appeal to me....		
c. I eat a balanced diet...........................		

These questions involve the kinds of moods you experience. Place a
check mark in the appropriate yes/no column:

	Yes	No
1. I have ups and downs................................		
2. I have more downs than ups.........................		

	Yes	No

3. I have periods when I am so <u>up</u> that I drive family and friends "nuts" with my frantic activity.........

4. Usually I am <u>down</u> with no experience of <u>ups</u> at all..

Indicate on the scale below the total percentage of your life that you have been depressed:

Always (100%)	Most of the Time (75%)	Sometimes (50% of my Life)	Seldom (25%)	Never Depressed Before Now

Do you exercise? Yes/No (circle one). If yes, indicate how often:

_____

_____

The following questions relate to the members of your family. Please try to indicate as much information as possible.

1. Are there other members of your family who experience these or dif-ferent problems?

Who?_____ What?_____ How Long?_____

_____ _____ _____

_____ _____ _____

2. Have any of the members of your family been treated by a psychol-ogist <u>or</u> a physician for psychological problems?

Who?_____ What?_____ How Long?_____

_____ _____ _____

_____ _____ _____

Please list the upsetting incidents <u>in your life</u>, as completely as you are able. Please be as exact as possible. Indicate the age of occurrence (i.e., when the incident happened to you).

                                                        Age of Occurrence

1. _____ _____

2. _____ _____

3. _____ _____

Age of Occurrence

4. _____ _____

5. _____ _____

6. _____ _____

7. _____ _____

8. _____ _____

Do you drink alcoholic beverages or use nonprescribed drugs (drugs not given to you by prescription from a physician)? Yes/No (circle one).

If you drink alcohol, please indicate how often and how much:

How much?_____ How often?_____

When did you start drinking (age)?_____

If you use nonprescribed drugs, please indicate what and how much:

What?_____ Amount?_____

Do you drink coffee or other caffeinated beverages? Yes/No (circle one). If yes, how much:

_____

Please list the things that make you <u>feel</u> good. Indicate in the yes/no column whether you do these things currently.

	Yes	No
1. _____		
2. _____		
3. _____		

Please list all of the people in your current support system and indicate their relationship to you.

Relationship   Relationship

1. _____ _____ 4. _____ _____

2. _____ _____ 5. _____ _____

3. _____ _____ 6. _____ _____

Post-Traumatic Stress Disorder

Please list those things in your life that you do to contribute to your problems or bad feelings:

1. _____   4. _____

2. _____   5. _____

3. _____   6. _____

Please list your hobbies and indicate in the yes/no column whether you continue to use them as diversions from your problems or for your own enjoyment:

		Yes	No*
1.	_____		
2.	_____		
3.	_____		
4.	_____		
5.	_____		

*(If no, indicate on the lines above, why not.)

Please answer the next two questions, only if you are a woman:

1. Have you ever noticed any changes in your mood as far as your monthly cycle is concerned? Yes/No (circle one). If not, please indicate whether you are willing to keep a daily calendar, recording your mood for three (3) months and compare it with your monthly cycle. Yes/No (circle one).

2. Are you currently taking birth-control pills? Yes/No (circle one). If yes, how long have you been taking them?

_____

Male and Female:

1. Do you or have you had any sexual difficulties or problems? Yes/No (circle one). If yes, what is the problem?

_____

   For how long?_____

2. Do you, or have you had, any physical problems? Yes/No (circle one). If yes, describe:

_____

Post-Traumatic Stress Disorder

Have you ever been told by a physician or psychologist that you had a
<u>physical ailment</u> that was related to a <u>psychological</u> condition?
Yes/No (circle one).

    If yes, what?_____

    How old were you?_____

    If yes, please describe your feelings about what you thought the
    physician or psychologist was saying to you:

    _____

    _____

Please indicate the <u>advantages</u> that your problem(s) give(s) you, when
you think about it/them in a <u>positive sense</u>:

1. _____

2. _____

3. _____

4. _____

5. _____

Please indicate what you hope to achieve from therapy:

1. _____

2. _____

3. _____

4. _____

5. _____

List <u>all</u> medications you are taking. Please include amount and reason:

	Medication	Amount	Reason
1.			
2.			
3.			
4.			
5.			

The following questions relate to your living arrangements and to your obligations and responsibilities (including how you spend your time):

Do you have a job? Yes/No (circle one). If yes, where?

_____

What do you do (duties, etc.)?_____

How many hours per week do you work?_____

Position title?_____

If you are now in school:

What school do you attend?_____

What year in school are you?_____

Do you like school? Yes/No (circle one). If not, why not?

_____

Indicate highest grade and/or degree completed:_____

What is/was your grade point average for highest grade/degree completed?

_____

Indicate major:_____

Below is a time schedule. Please indicate what you do during the hours of the day as closely as you can:

How many hours do you sleep at night, generally?_____

Time I typically get up in the morning is: Weekdays:_____

Weekends:_____

Time I typically go to bed at night is: Weekdays:_____

Weekends:_____

Schedule							
Time	Sun	Mon	Tues	Wed	Thurs	Fri	Sat
5:00-7:00 am							
8:00 am							

204

Time	Sun	Mon	Tues	Wed	Thurs	Fri	Sat
9:00 am							
10:00 am							
11:00 am							
noon							
1:00 pm							
2:00 pm							
3:00 pm							
4:00 pm							
5:00 pm							
6:00 pm							
7:00 pm							
8:00 pm							
9:00 pm							
10:00 pm							
After 10 pm							

Schedule (Continued)

Please describe your living situation. Do you live in a house or apartment? How many rooms, and so forth? What is it like?

_____

_____

_____

_____

Do you live alone? Yes/No (circle one). If yes, is this by choice? Yes/No (circle one).

If you do not live alone, how many people do you live with?_____

Do you consider the people you live with to be your friends?   Yes/No (circle one). If not, why?

_____

List the people living with you. Indicate in the yes/no column whether you regard them as supportive of you or as being a positive influence around you:

Name	Relationship	Age	Supportive?	
			Yes	No*

*If no, indicate on the lines above,
why you believe they are being nonsupportive.

Have you been in trouble with the law? Yes/No (circle one).

If yes, what was the trouble, and when did it occur?_____

_____

_____

What was the outcome?_____

Please list those events in your life which you regard as <u>failure experiences</u> or <u>big</u> mistakes you have made. Indicate the age at which you experienced it (them):

Events/Experiences	Age
1. _____	
2. _____	

Post-Traumatic Stress Disorder

Events/Experiences	Age
3. _____	_____
4. _____	_____
5. _____	_____

The following question has to do with grief experiences and losses in life. Please indicate what the loss was and at what age it occurred:

Losses	Age
1. _____	_____
2. _____	_____
3. _____	_____
4. _____	_____
5. _____	_____

Do you have problems with friends? Yes/No (circle one). If yes, what kinds of problems do you have?

_____

_____

Do you have problems with family members? Yes/No (circle one). If yes, who do you have problems with and what kinds of problems are they?

_____

_____

_____

_____

_____

_____

Please indicate on the scales below, in the appropriate area, the following:

I am guilt prone:

Always	Sometimes	Hardly Ever	Never

I am perfectionistic:

Always	Sometimes	Hardly Ever	Never

I lack self-esteem:

Always	Sometimes	Hardly Ever	Never

I am relatively independent from others:

Always	Sometimes	Hardly Ever	Never

I depend on others to help me out of my problem(s) or to make me feel better about myself:

Always	Sometimes	Hardly Ever	Never

People let me down:

Always	Sometimes	Hardly Ever	Never

I pay a lot of attention to my surroundings:

Always	Sometimes	Hardly Ever	Never

I have had good experiences with pets in my life:

Always	Sometimes	Hardly Ever	Never

When I am depressed, I feel lonely:

Always	Sometimes	Hardly Ever	Never

When I am depressed, I feel a remarkable decrease in my level of functioning:

Always	Sometimes	Hardly Ever	Never

I make an effort to have a sense of humor:

Always	Sometimes	Hardly Ever	Never

I have enough energy to do all the things I want to do:

Always	Sometimes	Hardly Ever	Never

Post-Traumatic Stress Disorder

I am a very pessimistic person:

_____
Always   Sometimes   Hardly Ever   Never

I try to please others and to do things for them:

_____
Always   Sometimes   Hardly Ever   Never

Marital status (circle one): Single/Married/Separated/Widowed/Divorced

   If married, name of spouse_____ Age_____

   Is spouse employed? Yes/No (circle one). If yes, where?

   _____

   Number of children?_____ Ages_____

   If separated, date of separation:_____

      Reason(s) for separation:_____

   If divorced, date of divorce:_____

      Reason(s) for divorce:_____

   If widowed, date of death of spouse:_____

      Cause(s) of death of spouse:_____

If ever married, how long married?_____

If married, separated, widowed, or divorced, is/was this your only
marriage? Yes/No (circle). If not, indicate the following:

Previous Spouse(s) Name	Your Age When Married	Length of Marriage	Reason for Termination of Marriage

Please list those things that you have stopped doing because of your problem(s) that you would like to start doing again, <u>now</u>:

1. _____

2. _____

3. _____

4. _____

List previous therapists you have seen; if a diagnosis was made regarding you, please include it, as well:

	Therapist	Address	Date(s) Seen	Diagnosis
1.				
2.				
3.				

Have you been hospitalized during your lifetime? Yes/No (circle one).

    If yes, specify below:

	Reason for Hospitalization	Physician	Date(s)	How Long?
1.				
2.				
3.				
4.				

Specify, as completely as you can, all medical conditions previously diagnosed:

	Condition	Date(s) of Condition	Present Now?	
1.			Yes	No
2.			Yes	No
3.			Yes	No
4.			Yes	No

                                                (circle one)

Please list all jobs/employment you have had (if necessary, use a separate sheet of paper):

	Position	Employer	How Long?	Reason(s) for Termination
1.				
2.				
3.				
4.				
5.				
6.				
7.				
8.				
9.				

When not in school, have you had times in which you were unemployed? Yes/No (circle). If yes, list dates of unemployment and reason(s):

	Dates of Unemployment	Reason(s)
1.		
2.		
3.		

Have you ever quit a job suddenly and for little or no reason? Yes/No (circle one). If yes, describe:

_____

_____

Have you ever been fired from a job? Yes/No (circle one). If yes, please describe:

_____

_____

_____

Post-Traumatic Stress Disorder

If you are <u>older</u> than 15 years of age, please answer the following:

		Yes	No
1.	Before I turned 15 years of age, I often skipped school...		
2.	I was expelled from school for misbehavior......... If yes, age(s) of expulsion:_____		
3.	I was arrested or sent to juvenile court for delinquency or for my misbehavior.................. If yes, age(s):_____		
4.	I ran away from home and stayed out all night at <u>least</u> twice while I was living in my parent(s)' or foster home <u>or</u> ran away once and didn't go back home.. If yes, age(s):_____		
5.	I told lies <u>a lot</u> when I was a child (before I was 15 years old)...................................		
6.	I forced someone to have sex with me before I was 15..		
7.	I was drunk a lot and abused drugs before I was 15 years old.......................................		
8.	I stole things when no one was around before I was 15..		
9.	I stole things regardless of whether anyone was around before I was 15.............................. If yes to #8 and/or #9, give age(s):_____		
10.	I purposely vandalized or destroyed property before I was 15.. If yes, give age(s):_____		
11.	Teachers told me or my parent(s) that my grades in school were too low to reflect my intelligence or IQ..		
12.	I broke a lot of rules at home and at school before I was 15..		
13.	I started a lot of fights when I was younger (before the age of 15)................................ If yes, give age(s):_____		
14.	I used a weapon in a couple of fights..............		
15.	I was physically abusive or cruel to animals before I was 15....................................		

	Yes	No

16. I was physically abusive or cruel to other people before I was 15.................................

17. I intentionally set fires before I was 15..........

Have you ever been in a court before? Yes/No (circle one).

    If yes, describe the circumstances:_____

_____

_____

Have you ever been sued? Yes/No (circle one).

    If yes, how many times?_____

    If yes, describe the circumstances:_____

_____

_____

Have you ever sued anyone else? Yes/No (circle one).

    If yes, how many times?_____

    If yes, describe the circumstances:_____

_____

_____

Do you have difficulties with your neighbors, boss, co-workers, and so on? Yes/No (circle one).

    If yes, who and why:_____

_____

_____

Have you ever had any accidents? Yes/No (circle one).

    If yes, how many?_____

    If yes, describe any accidents you have had:_____

_____

_____

_____

_____

Have you had problems handling money? Yes/No (circle one).

    If yes, describe the problems:_____

    _____

    _____

Have you had any problems with credit (either having difficulty obtaining it or having credit revoked?) Yes/No (circle one).

    If yes, describe:_____

    _____

Have you ever been evicted from your home or apartment? Yes/No (circle one).

    If yes, describe the circumstances:_____

    _____

    _____

    _____

Please indicate how filling out this questionnaire has affected you:

_____

_____

_____

Also, in filling out this questionnaire, you have/have not (circle one) had any clues about what you could do to help yourself with your problem(s). If you have not had any clues, please re-read the questionnaire and see if you notice any. Then, try to fill out the following:

List those things you would like to try to change (possibilities to include in your life):

1. _____

2. _____

3. _____

4. _____

Indicate any other possible changes that might help you alter your lifestyle and help you improve your mood or problem(s):

1. _____

2. _____

3. _____

4. _____

214

In the space below, please include any other information about yourself that you think would be helpful in understanding you and your
problem(s):

_____

_____

_____

_____

Please look back over the questionnaire, decide if you have omitted
anything; if you have, please add it. If you ran out of room on an
item, please use a separate sheet of paper - title the paper with the
question you are continuing to answer. Thank you.

_____

This is the end of the questionnaire. One of the things that many
people have discovered in filling out this instrument is that significant events in their lives are often forgotten while filling it out
and only occur to them _later_ in their therapy, or at other times.
Often, people do not include some things in this questionnaire
because they think those things are unimportant. Many times they do
not wish to include some information because they are, at that point
in time, lacking trust in their therapist and are making decisions
about whether to tell the therapist some things about themselves.
Often, when the relationship in therapy becomes more comfortable,
people decide they want to add things to this questionnaire. If this
happens to you, please ask to have the questionnaire back and add the
information that is remembered later. Thank you for filling it out.
The information you have provided may be helpful in helping you with
your problem(s).

_____

AUTHOR INDEX

Author Index

Achenbach, T. M., 98-99, 125
Adams-Tucker, C., 94, 97-98, 117, 125
Akhtar, S., 137-138, 152
Alexander, H., 102-103, 114, 133
Allen, I. M., 9, 11, 16, 52
Alter-Reid, K., 118, 122, 125
Alvarez, M., 114, 129, 141, 153
Ambonetti, A., 54
American Bar Association, 193
American Medical Association, 163-164, 166
American Psychiatric Association, 2, 7, 10, 13, 26, 39, 40-41, 49, 52, 63, 72-73, 75, 77, 87, 92, 105, 111-112, 125, 137, 152, 189
Andersen, B. L., 57
Anderson, S. C., 96-99, 125
Andreasen, N. C., 10-11, 15-19, 23-24, 52
Archibald, H. C., 11, 15-16, 24, 52
Arnold, A. L., 9, 11, 23, 25-26, 50, 52
Arnold, L. E., 94, 127
Arthur, R. J., 11, 15, 22, 25-26, 45, 52, 57
Athavale, V. B., 94, 131
Atkinson, R. M., 4, 7, 9, 16, 19, 21, 26, 43, 52, 59, 85-86, 89, 138, 142-143, 145, 147, 150

Bach, C. M., 96-99, 125
Bachman, L., 138, 154
Bagley, C., 104, 125
Bailey, J. E., 21, 23, 43, 50, 52
Baritz, L., 80, 87
Barlow, D. H., 64, 72, 117, 126
Baruch, E., 11, 23, 56
Baum, A., 119, 127
Beasley, M., 143, 152
Behar, D., 140, 152
Beigel, A., 4, 7, 11, 15, 21-22, 52, 58
Beilke, R., 98-99, 128
Ben, R., 11, 16, 45, 53, 56
Benbenishty, R., 11, 59
Bender, L., 91-92, 94, 96, 125-126
Bender, M. E., 118, 130
Benedek, E. D., 4, 7, 11, 52, 91, 112, 126
Benedikt, R., 140, 152
Berliner, L., 122, 127
Berren, M. R., 4, 7, 11, 15, 21-22, 52
Bhatt, S. C., 94, 131
Biaggio, M. K., 121, 133
Blakey, W. J., 193
Blanchard, E. B., 117, 126
Blank, A. S., 9-10, 19, 21, 23, 42, 53, 56, 58-59, 85, 87, 89, 138, 147, 152, 155
Blau, A., 91, 94, 96, 125
Bleich, A., 9, 11, 14, 31, 40, 45, 55, 59, 138, 155
Blitz, R., 137, 146, 156

219

Bloch, A. M., 23, 53
Blumberg, M., 143, 152
Boatman, B., 96, 126
Boehnlein, J. K., 11, 16, 45, 53
Boon, C., 103, 114, 133
Borus, J., 143, 152
Boulanger, G., 9, 16, 19, 53, 78, 88
Bourne, P. G., 79, 87-88
Boydstun, J. A., 10-11, 20-21, 60
Braceland, F. J., 9-10, 53
Branch, G., 94, 126
Brandon, S., 102, 132
Brandt, R., 94, 126
Braun, B., 103, 132
Breslau, N., 9, 11, 53
Brett, E. A., 9, 42, 53, 56, 115, 130
Brewster, T., 84, 88
Bridges, M., 10, 19, 54
Briere, J., 100, 102-104, 115, 126
Bromberg, W., 53
Brooks, B., 104-105, 133
Broun, K. S., 193
Browne, A., 92-93, 96, 100, 104, 114, 126
Browning, D. H., 96, 126
Buck, C., 102, 121, 128
Buckhart, B., 149, 152
Burgess, A. W., 10-11, 19, 21-22, 42, 45, 53, 94, 107-108, 126, 138, 141, 152
Burke, J., 143, 152
Burr, W., 137, 146, 156
Burstein, A., 45, 53
Burton, L., 94, 126
Butler, R. W., 57
Byrne, K., 53

Cacioppo, J. T., 57
Caddell, J. M., 118, 130
Calestro, K., 94, 127
Call, J. D., 106, 128
Canas, R., 145, 154
Canteen, W., 9, 55
Caplan, G., 117, 126
Carlson, R. L., 180, 193
Carroll, E. M., 14-15, 54, 124, 128
Cavenar, J. O., 10, 60, 148, 152
Centers for Disease Control, 142, 152
Chen, J. J., 58, 140, 155
Christenson, R. M., 9, 16, 53
Christian, W., 149, 152

Claypatch, C., 102, 129
Coburn, K., 13, 23, 45, 60
Cohen, J. A., 96-99, 131, 137-138, 153
Cole, C. F., 104, 134
Conte, J. R., 122, 124, 127
Corcoran, J. F. T., 9, 11, 53
Cornfield, R. B., 10, 16, 45, 54
Corson, J. A., 9, 11, 16, 54
Courtois, C. A., 100, 102-105, 115, 127
Cowley, R. A., 15, 18, 58
Cross, H. J., 79, 88
Cullen, M. R., 19, 58, 145, 155

Damlouji, N., 143, 153
Darwin, M. R., 96, 134
Davidson, L. M., 119, 127
Davis, G. C., 9, 11, 53
Deale, S., 4, 7, 9, 16, 26, 52
DeFrancis, V., 94, 96-98, 127
Dent, O. F., 11, 59
Devinney, L., 79, 89
de Young, M., 104, 127
Diamond, B., 137-138, 153
Dickinson, E., iii
Dillon, H., 11, 13, 15-16, 20-22, 56
Dimsdale, J. E., 11, 54
Distad, L. J., 11, 14-15, 56, 103, 113-115, 120-121, 123, 130
DiVasto, P., 102-103, 128
Dixon, K. N., 94, 127
Domash, M., 139-140, 153
Donahoe, C. P., Jr., 14-15, 54
Donaldson, M. A., 102-103, 113, 120-121, 123, 127
Dunn, C. G., 18, 54
Dutton, D. E., 96, 134

Early, E., 138, 153
Eaton, W. W., 11, 16, 54
Edelbrock, C., 98-99, 125
Edgar, M., 104, 134
Enoch, D., 11, 20, 56, 137, 154
Erichsen, J. E., 74, 88
Erikson, K. T., 11, 17, 54
Erlinder, C., 137, 153
Eth, S., 106, 127
Ettedgui, E., 10, 19, 54
Everstine, D. S., 92-93, 127
Everstine, L., 92-93, 127

Fagan, J., 103, 127
Fairbank, J. A., 50, 54, 117-118, 130-
131, 149-150, 153-154
Faravelli, C., 54
Federal Rules of Evidence, 174-185,
193
Feldman-Summers, S., 104, 134
Ferenczi, S., 94, 127
Ferguson, J., 143, 153
Figley, C. R., 73, 87-88
Finkelhor, D., 11, 23, 54, 92-93, 96,
100, 104-105, 114, 126,
128
Fitzsimmons, J. T., 9, 19, 21, 52
Fleck, J., 11, 16, 45, 53, 56
Flicker, D., 149, 153
Fonnesu, F., 54
Forbes, L. M., 94, 128
Forward, S., 102, 121, 128
Fowler, D., 138, 154
Fox, S. S., 11, 19, 21, 45, 54
Foy, D. W., 14-15, 54, 124, 128
Frances, A., 68, 72
Francois, R., 138, 154
Frankl, V. E., 82, 88
Fredrickson, R. H., 11, 16, 45, 56
Friedman, M. J., 9, 11, 16, 54
Friedrich, W. N., 98-99, 128
Fromuth, M. E., 105, 128
Frye, J. S., 9, 54

Gagnon, J., 91, 128
Gallers, J., 14-15, 54
Gallops, M. S., 9, 56, 115, 130
Garb, R., 9, 14, 31, 40, 45, 55, 59,
138, 155
Gardner, R., 102-103, 113, 120-
121, 123, 127
Gebhard, P. H., 91, 130
Gelinas, D. J., 112-113, 128
George, J. A., 186-191, 193
Gerardi, R. J., 117-119, 126, 134
Giaretto, H., 120, 128
Gibbs, M. S., 118, 122, 125
Gislason, I. L., 106, 128
Gladstone, T., 106, 133
Gold, E. R., 122, 128
Golden, G., 77, 88
Gomes-Schwartz, B., 99, 128
Goodwin, D. W., 40-41, 55
Goodwin, J., 102-103, 116, 128,
132, 138, 153

Gorcey, M., 11, 58
Gornick, J., 11, 20-21, 57
Gorsuch, R. L., 119, 133
Gough, H., 149-150, 153
Goulston, K. J., 11, 59
Greenfeld, H., 11, 23, 56
Griffith, S., 96-99, 125
Grinker, R. R., 78-79, 88
Groesbeck, C. J., 9-10, 55
Groth, A. N., 94, 108, 126
Grugett, A. E., 91-92, 126
Grupper, D., 11, 59, 138, 155
Guyon, R., 91, 129
Guze, S. B., 40-41, 55
Gynther, M., 149, 152

Haley, S. A., 11, 31, 55
Hall, R. C. W., 11, 19, 21, 55
Halperin, G., 11, 20, 56, 137, 154
Hamilton, J. D. V., 9, 55
Harrison, P. A., 102, 129
Hartman, C. R., 94, 107-108, 126
Hartmann, E., 137, 146-147, 153,
156
Hathaway, S. E., 119, 129
Hefez, A., 11, 20, 56, 137, 153-154
Henderson, D. J., 91, 129
Henderson, J., 91, 129
Henderson, R. G., 4, 7, 9, 16, 26,
52, 138, 142-143, 145, 147,
152
Hendin, H., 9, 13, 55, 141, 153
Herman, J. L., 96, 98, 102-104, 121,
123-124, 129
Hillman, R. G., 11, 55
Hirschman, L., 96, 129
Hocking, F., 141, 153
Hoffman, B. F., 12, 16, 18, 21, 43,
55
Hogben, G., 10, 16, 45, 54
Hoiberg, A., 11, 19, 21, 25, 55
Holmes, O., Jr., 161, 166
Holmstrom, L. L., 10-11, 19, 21-22,
42, 45, 53, 94, 126, 138,
141, 152
Horowitz, M. J., 14-18, 20-22, 24-
26, 55, 75-77, 82, 87-88,
99, 114-115, 117, 120-121,
128-129, 140-141, 153
Hyler, S., 147, 153

Imwinkelried, E. J., 180, 193
Isaacs, S., 96, 129

Jackson, T. L., 11, 45, 55
Jaffe, A. C., 94, 134
James, J., 104, 129
Jefferies, J., 143, 154
Jelinek, J. M., 41, 56
Jones, D. P. H., 120-122, 129
Jurich, A. P., 82, 88
Justice, B., 130
Justice, R., 130

Kalkarni, B. S., 94, 131
Kaltreider, N., 114, 129
Kapp, F. T., 11, 15, 60, 143, 156
Kardiner, A., 142, 146, 154
Karls, W., 11, 16, 45, 56
Karpinski, E., 91, 96, 102, 133
Katan, A., 103, 130
Kaufman, I., 96, 130
Keane, T. M., 50, 54, 117-119, 130-
        131, 134, 149-150, 153-154
Kemph, J. P., 91-92, 135
Kiev, A., 191, 194
Kinsey, A. C., 91, 130
Kinzie, J. D., 11, 16, 45, 53, 56
Kionka, E. J., 180, 193
Klajner-Diamond, H., 94, 98, 131
Kleinhesselink, R. R., 79, 88
Kluft, R., 103, 107-108, 130
Kocsis, J., 68, 72
Kolb, L. C., 16, 56, 117, 126, 137,
        140, 148-149, 152, 154
Kormos, H. R., 82, 88
Kovach, J., 104, 113, 130
Krieger, M., 94, 132
Krystal, H., 138, 141, 143, 145, 148,
        154

LaBarre, W., 82, 88
Lacey, G., 106, 130
Lachenmeyer, J. R., 118, 122, 125
LaGuardia, R., 138, 154
Langmade, C. J., 104, 130
Larose, L., 117, 135
Laufer, R. S., 9, 56, 115, 130
Lavie, P., 11, 20, 56, 137, 153-154
Lazarus, R. S., 77, 88
LeBaron, D., 94, 98, 131
Lempert, R. O., 194

Leopold, R. L., 11, 13, 15-16, 20-
        22, 56
Lerer, B., 9, 14, 31, 40, 45, 55
Levav, I. L., 11, 23, 56
Lewis, M., 94, 130
Lifton, R. J., 9, 13, 15, 45, 56, 115,
        130
Lindberg, F. H., 11, 14-15, 56, 103,
        113-115, 120-121, 123, 130
Lindemann, E., 117, 130
Lindy, J. D., 11, 45, 56
Lipkin, J. O., 9, 19, 21, 23, 42, 56
Lister, E. D., 56
Loftus, E., 57, 140, 154
Loftus, T., 140, 154
Lokeshwar, M. R., 94, 131
Long, C., 70-72
Long, D. M., 11, 15-16, 24, 52
Lopez-Ibor, J., 145, 154
Louisell, D. W., 194
Luisada, P., 143, 154
Lukianowicz, N., 96, 131
Lumry, A. E., 102, 129
Lushene, R. E., 119, 133
Lusk, R., 92-93, 98, 131
Lyons, J. A., 117-119, 134

MacFarlane, K., 91, 93, 131
Maisch, H., 94, 96, 131
Malloy, P. F., 117, 131, 150, 154
Malone, P. T., 11, 19, 21, 55
Maltbie, A. A., 9, 16, 53, 148, 152
Mannarino, A. P., 96-99, 131
Martin, C. E., 91, 130
Martzke, J. S., 57
Masson, J. M., 91, 131
Massoth, N. A., 118, 122, 125
Mayfield, D., 138, 154
McCaffrey, R. J., 50, 54, 149, 153
McCall-Perez, F., 11, 58
McCarthy, T., 102-103, 128
McCaughey, B. G., 11, 19, 21, 25,
        55
McCausland, M. B., 94, 107-108,
        126
McElhaney, J. W., 194
McFarland, R. E., 58, 140, 155
McFarlane, A. C., 11, 16, 57
McKenna, G. J., 11, 15, 22, 26, 45,
        52, 57
McKinley, T. C., 119, 129
McKinnon, J., 9, 60, 138, 156

McMahon, P. O., 103, 127
McNeil, G., 65, 68-69, 72
Meek, C. L., 4, 7
Mehta, M. N., 94, 131
Meier, J. H., 94, 133
Meiselman, K. C., 97-98, 100, 102,
    104-105, 121, 131
Metz, L., 137, 153
Meyerding, J., 104, 129
Mian, M., 94, 98, 131
Mikulincer, M., 11, 59
Miller, C., 11, 16, 24, 52
Miller, L. C., 97, 131
Millstein, K., 143, 152
Modlin, H. C., 10, 15-17, 20-23, 25,
    44, 57, 63, 72, 159-160,
    164, 166
Monahan, J., 57
Mrazek, D. A., 93, 100, 131
Mrazek, P. B., 92-93, 100, 131
Mueser, K. T., 57
Muse, M., 22, 24, 57
Mutalipassi, L. R., 16, 56

Nadelson, C. C., 11, 20-22, 57, 94,
    132
Nakashima, I. I., 93-94, 96, 131-132
Nash, J., 148, 152
Nathan, P., 140, 155
Nemiah, J., 66, 72
Newman, C. J., 11, 13, 57, 106, 132
Niederland, W., 141, 154
Nielson, T., 94, 132
Norman, E. M., 124, 132
Notman, M. T., 11, 20-22, 57
Nurcombe, B., 106, 133

Oppenheimer, R., 102, 132
Ostroff, R., 42, 53

Palmer, R. L., 102, 132
Pankratz, L., 59, 138, 155
Paxton, R., 94, 126
Peck, A., 94, 96, 130
Peele, R., 143, 154
Peters, J. J., 93, 97-98, 132
Peters, S. D., 104, 132
Peterson, C., 122, 132
Petretic-Jackson, P. A., 11, 45, 55
Phillips, M., 137-138, 142, 144, 154
Pina, G., III, 9, 57
Pines, A. M., 104, 133

Pittard, E., 143, 154
Pollinger, A., 9, 13, 55, 141, 153
Pomeroy, W. B., 91, 130
Powers, R., 107-108, 126
Prosser, W., 158, 166
Putnam, F., 103, 132
Pynoos, R. S., 106, 127

Quevillon, R. P., 11, 45, 55

Rabinovitch, R. D., 96, 132
Raifman, L., 137, 142, 146-148, 155
Ramsay, R., 104, 125
Rangell, L., 11, 17, 20-21, 58
Ravenscroft, K., 11, 58
Reid, W. H., 58
Reno, R., 14-15, 54
Resnick, P., 137-138, 155
Rhinehart, J. W., 102, 132
Ries, R., 137-138, 142, 144, 154
Riggs, R. S., 94, 96, 132
Robins, L., 78, 89
Rodriguez-Gamazo, M., 145, 154
Rogers, E., 96, 134
Rogers, R., 138, 145, 149-150, 155
Rome, H. P., 58
Rose, D. S., 11, 58
Rosenfeld, A. A., 94, 132
Ross, D. R., 9, 16, 53
Rothschild, A. J., 11, 25-26, 58
Rueger, D. B., 124, 128
Runtz, M., 103-104, 126
Russell, D. E. H., 103, 124, 129, 132.
Russell, W., 140, 155

Sachs, R., 103, 132
Saltzburg, S. A., 194
Santiago, J. M., 11, 58
Sarrell, P. M., 94, 130
Sauzier, M., 99, 128
Schacter, D., 140, 155
Schatzow, E., 103, 121, 123, 129
Scherl, D. J., 11, 19, 21, 45, 54
Schnaper, N., 15, 18, 58
Schneiderman, C. K., 9, 11, 16, 54
Schottenfeld, R. S., 19, 58, 145, 155
Schuerman, J. R., 124, 127
Schwarzwald, J., 11, 59
Scrignar, C. B., 9, 14, 16, 18, 58
Scurfield, R. M., 9, 19, 21, 23, 42,
    56, 58, 138, 155
Sedney, M. A., 104-105, 133

Seligman, M. E. P., 122, 132
Senior, N., 106, 133
Sessarego, A., 54
Shatan, C. F., 9, 11, 20-21, 58, 77, 89
Shaw, V. L., 94, 133
Shealy, C. N., 22, 58
Sheff, A. G., 9, 19, 21, 52
Sherry, S., 137, 146, 156
Shore, J. H., 11, 58
Sierles, F. S., 58, 140, 142, 155
Sigal, J. J., 11, 16, 54, 118, 122, 125
Silbert, M. H., 104, 133
Silver, R. L., 103, 114, 133
Silver, S. M., 10-11, 20, 23, 26, 59
Singer, M. T., 10-11, 15, 20-21, 59
Singer, P., 9, 13, 55, 141, 153
Sipprelle, R. C., 124, 128
Sloane, P., 91, 96, 102, 133
Smith, G., 138, 154
Smith, J. R., 10, 59, 118, 133
Solomon, G. F., 115, 129
Solomon, Z., 11, 59, 138, 155
Sonnenberg, S. M., 10, 59, 87, 89
Soria, J., 145, 154
Sparr, L. F., 4, 7, 9, 16, 19, 21, 26, 43, 52, 59, 85-86, 89, 138-140, 142-143, 145, 147, 152-153, 155
Spiegel, D., 140, 155
Spiegel, J. P., 79, 88
Spielberger, C. D., 119, 133
Spiro, H., 137-138, 142, 155
Spitzer, R. L., 118, 133, 147, 153
Star, S., 79, 89
Steele, B. F., 102-103, 114, 133
Stern, G. M., 11, 25, 59, 138, 155
Stockton, R. A., 9, 54
Stone, M. H., 30, 59
Stones, S. M. H., 103, 114, 133
Stouffer, S., 79, 89
Suchman, E., 79, 89
Summers, H. G., 80, 89
Summit, R. C., 96, 133
Swanson, L., 121, 133
Symonds, M., 138, 155

Tagiuri, C., 94, 96, 130
Talbott, J. A., 10, 59, 87, 89
Tarek, D., 94, 134
Tatum, E. L., 11, 58
Taylor, M. A., 58, 140, 155

Taylor, S. E., 13, 59, 77, 89
Tennant, C. C., 11, 59
Terr, L. C., 4, 106-107, 112, 117, 120, 133-134, 140-141, 155
Thompson, G. N., 15, 18-19, 60
Tilelli, J. A., 94, 134
Tisza, V., 94, 126
Titchener, J. L., 11, 15, 60, 138, 141, 143, 145, 156
Trimble, M. R., 71-72, 89
Trocki, K., 124, 129
Tsai, M., 102, 104, 114, 122, 134
Tuddenham, R. D., 11, 15-16, 24, 52
Tufts' New England Medical Center, 96-99, 134

Ulman, R. B., 9, 13, 55, 141, 153
Urquiza, A. J., 98-99, 128
Ursano, R. J., 10-11, 20-21, 60

Van Buskirk, S. S., 104, 134
van der Kolk, B. A., 22, 60, 137, 146, 156
Van Dyke, C., 9, 60, 138, 156
Vera, E., 11, 16-18, 22, 26, 44, 60
Vollmer, W. M., 11, 58

Wagner, N. N., 102, 104, 114, 122, 134
Walker, J. I., 9-10, 16, 53, 60
Ward, N., 137-138, 142, 144, 154
Waterman, J., 92-93, 98, 131
Watts, D. L., 100, 102-103, 115, 127
Webb, T., 54
Webb, W., 70-72
Webster's New World Dictionary, 167, 186, 194
Wehrspann, W., 94, 98, 131
Weinfeld, M., 11, 16, 54
Weisenberg, M., 11, 59
Weiss, J., 96, 134
Weissman, H. N., 60
Welner, N., 141, 153
West, A. N., 9, 11, 16, 54
West, L. J., 13, 23, 45, 60
Wheatley, R. D., 10-11, 20-21, 60
White, R. A. F., 9, 19, 21, 52
Wilcox, F. A., 84, 89
Wilkinson, C. B., 11, 16-18, 22, 26, 44-45, 60

224

Williams, J. B., 118, 133
Williams, R., 79, 89
Williams, T., 41, 56, 79, 89, 120, 134
Wilmer, H. A., 11, 16, 60, 139, 156
Wilner, M., 114, 129
Winder, C., 94, 98, 131
Wolfe, D. A., 117, 134-135
Wolfe, J., 117-119, 134
Wolfe, V. V., 117, 134-135

Yates, A., 91, 135
Yorukoglu, A., 91-92, 135

Zackson, H., 11, 20-21, 57
Zakus, G., 93-94, 131-132
Zilberg, N., 9, 60, 138, 156
Zimering, R. T., 118, 130
Ziskin, J., 42, 46, 60-61

SUBJECT INDEX

Subject Index*

Abandonment fears, 144, 148

Abuse of psychoactive substances, 27, 30, 40-42, 79-81, 84, 101, 103-104, 108, 138-140, 142, 147, 150

    alcohol, 41-42, 140, 142, 147, 150

    drugs, 79-81, 140, 142, 147, 150

    SAV, 101, 103-104, 108, 138-139

Abuse, sexual, 91-124

    adults abused as children - effects, 100-105, 109-124

    child/adolescent abuse - effects, 91-100, 105-112, 116-117, 119-120

Academic history, 23, 71

Academic problems - child/adolescent SAV, 94-96, 99, 108

Acting-out behavior - SAV, 94-98, 101, 108, 111-112, 117, 123 (see also pages 45-46)

Acute combat reaction, 82

Acute PTSD, 2, 143

Adaptation to stress, 26, 77, 161

Adjustment Disorder, 26-28, 30, 39, 64-65, 73

Admissibility of evidence, 184-186

Adolescence or Childhood Differential Diagnosis (see Childhood or Adolescence - Differential Diagnosis)

Adolescent antisocial behavior, 27, 30, 45-56, 94-99, 109, 117

Adolescent sexual abuse (see Abuse, sexual; child/adolescent abuse - effects)

Adult Differential Diagnosis (see Differential Diagnosis - Adults)

Adults, sexually abused as children - effects, 100-105, 109-124

Affect - Problems with, 67-68, 77, 106, 110, 140

    restriction/constriction of, 77, 106, 110, 140

Affection-seeking behavior - child/adolescent SAV, 94-95

Affective difficulties - SAV, 94-97, 100-102, 105, 114-115, 117-118

Affective Disorders (see Mood Disorders)

Age of victim, 141

Aggressive behavior - child/adolescent SAV, 97, 99

Aggressivity, 17, 43, 97, 99, 109

---

*ABBREVIATIONS: PTSD - Post-Traumatic Stress Disorder
                      SAV - Sexual Abuse Victims

Aging, 38, 41
  later-life symptoms (multiple) - invariably due to physical illness, 41, 49
Agoraphobia, 65-66
Alcohol abuse, 41-42, 103-104, 108, 140, 142, 147, 150
  adult SAV, 103-104
  child/adolescent SAV, 108
Alcohol intolerance, 70
Alcoholics Anonymous, 104, 113
Alexithymia, 141
Alienation, 101-104, 110, 144, 150
Alternatives to Sexual Abuse organization, 4
Ambivalent feelings - child/adolescent, 114, 122
Amnesia, 29, 38, 69, 101, 103, 110, 114, 140, 147
Anger, 17, 43, 78, 83, 94-95, 97, 99, 105, 110, 112, 114, 121-122, 150
  adult SAV, 105, 110, 121-122, 150
  child/adolescent SAV, 94-95, 97, 99, 105, 110, 112, 114, 121-122
Anhedonia, 150
Animal cruelty - child/adolescent, 45
Animal phobia, 28
Anniversary reactions, 69, 109, 148
Anorexia Nervosa, 30, 33
Anorgasmia - SAV, 102, 104
Anticipation of disaster, 22-23, 81, 160
Antisocial behavior, 27, 30, 36, 40-41, 43, 45-46, 63, 85-86, 94-99, 101, 108-109, 111-112, 117, 123
  child/adolescent, 27, 30, 36, 45-46, 99, 109, 117
  SAV, 94-99, 101, 108-109, 111-112, 117, 123
Antisocial Personality Disorder, 17, 27, 30, 40-46, 48-49, 142, 150
Antiwar sentiment - Vietnam conflict, 79-81
Anxiety, 26, 46, 70, 75-76, 94-97, 101-102, 104-107, 111-113, 115-119, 146-147, 150

Anxiety *(Continued)*
  child/adolescent, 94-97, 106-107, 111-112, 116-117
Anxiety Disorders, 1-4, 9-26, 28, 30, 33, 36, 40, 42-45, 50, 63-67, 70-71, 73-79, 82-87, 92, 94-95, 105-124, 137-151, 157-165, 191
  child/adolescent, 27-28, 30, 33, 36, 94-95
  Generalized Anxiety Disorder, 63-65, 118, 160
  Obsessive-Compulsive Disorder, 28
  Panic Disorder, 28, 36, 63-67
  PTSD, 1-4, 9-26, 36, 40, 42-45, 50, 63-64, 70-71, 73-79, 82-87, 92, 105-124, 137-151, 157-165, 191
  Simple phobia, 28
Anxiety Disorders of Childhood or Adolescence, 27-28, 30, 33, 36, 94-95
  Avoidant Disorder, 27
  Separation Anxiety Disorder, 28, 30, 33, 36, 94-95
Anxiety neurosis *(see Generalized Anxiety Disorder; Panic Disorder)*
Anxious expectation, 64
Appetite disturbances *(see Eating Disorders)*
Apprehension, 64-66
Arousal *(see Autonomic arousal)*
Artwork - child SAV, 120-121
Assessment, 2-3, 11-51, 63-71, 74, 78-79, 81-82, 84, 86, 91-124, 137-144, 147, 149-151, 157, 159-164, 190, 197-215
  bereavement, 30-31, 40, 69
  caffeine, 42
  Child Behavior Checklist, 98-99
  concurrent disorders, 3, 16-17, 143-144
  confounding factors/disorders, 14-17, 32-49, 160
  disability, 157, 160, 162-164
  extent of stressors, 12-13
  Global Assessment of Functioning Scale, 12
  grief, 30-31, 40, 144

Assessment *(Continued)*
  meaning of stressors, 13-14, 81-82, 137, 140-141, 143-144
  military history, 23, 71, 86, 138-141, 143-144
  Minnesota Multiphasic Personality Inventory, 46, 50, 119, 149-151
  multiple stressors, 2, 12, 14, 21-26, 39, 107, 143, 151
  noncompliance with, 15, 44-45, 47-48
  patient history, 13, 23, 43, 71, 120, 141, 151
  physical injuries, 11, 13, 18, 24-25, 29, 137, 139-140, 159, 163
  predisposing factors, 13, 19-24, 28, 32-39, 47-49
  predisposition, 19-24, 36, 74, 78-79, 86, 157, 161-162
  pre-existing conditions/vulnerabilities, 16, 18-24, 26, 28, 32-39, 47-49, 161-162
  premorbid personality, 16, 23-24, 35, 120, 143-144, 161-162
  psychoactive substance abuse, 27, 30, 40-42, 63, 65, 84, 103-104, 108, 117, 140, 142, 147, 150
  Self-Evaluation of Difficulties Questionnaire, 50-51, 197-215
  Severity of Psychosocial Stressors Scale, 12
  sexual abuse, 91-124
    adults abused as children, 100-105, 109-124
    child/adolescent SAV, 91-100, 105-112, 116-117, 119-120
    stress-related diagnosis, 26-30
    testing, 12, 46, 50, 97-99, 117-119, 149-151, 190
Associations to event, 1, 14, 45, 75-76, 106-109, 114-115, 119, 143
Atrocities - witness of, 11, 25, 83, 138-141, 143, 147

Attention-Deficit Hyperactivity Disorder, 30, 32, 36
Attention problems (see Concentration difficulties)
Attorneys, roles of, 15-17, 44, 71, 86, 157, 166-193
Authority figures, problems with, 43, 81-82, 103-104, 108, 120, 138-139, 150
  child/adolescent SAV, 103-104, 108, 138-139
Autonomic arousal, 64, 75, 77-78, 108, 110-112, 137, 149
Autonomic lability, 18
Avoidance behavior, 1, 18, 63, 73, 77, 94, 96, 99, 101-102, 104-105, 109-110, 112, 114-115, 119, 143, 150
  adult SAV, 101-102, 104, 109-110, 112
  child/adolescents, 94, 96, 99, 109-110, 112
Avoidant Disorder of Childhood or Adolescence, 27
Avoidant Personality Disorder, 36

Battering (see Spousal abuse - SAV)
Battle fatigue, 74
Battle stress, 10
Bedwetting (see Enuresis)
Behavioral changes (see Post-trauma changes)
Bereavement, 30-31, 40, 69
Betrayal feelings, 22, 117
Bipolar Disorder, 35, 67-68
Birth of sibling as stressor, 33
Blaming, 43, 76-79, 151
  others, 43, 76-77
  the victim, 78-79, 151
Borderline Personality Disorder, 22, 27, 30, 118
Brain syndromes (see Organic brain syndromes)
Brainwashing - child/adolescent SAV, 107-108
Brecksville PTSD Inventory, 118
Brief Reactive Psychosis, 27-28, 30, 34-35, 63, 68, 86
Briquet's syndrome (see Somatization Disorder)
Burden of proof, 158
"But for" theory, 162

Caffeine, 42
Calling of witnesses, 177
Captive, being held, 11, 38, 84, 138, 144-145
Cardiac symptoms, 66
Careful questioning (*see* Interviewing techniques)
Case scenarios, 1-4, 65-71, 138-140, 147-148, 159, 161, 163
  automobile accident, 1-2, 65, 68-69, 148, 163
  burns, 163
  Chowchilla school-bus kidnapping, 3-4
  concussion, 70-71
  explosion, 161
  Generalized Anxiety Disorder, 65
  Major Depression, 1-2, 68-69
  Panic Disorder, 66-67
  PTSD, 1-2, 68-69
  product liability, 159
  Vietnam experiences, 138-140, 147
  work-related accident, 66-67, 70-71
CAT scan, 71
Cerebral concussion (*see* Concussion)
"Chain of events" concept, 23
Changes in behavior (*see* Post-trauma changes)
Child sexual abuse, 32, 91-100, 105-112, 116-117, 119-120
Child Behavior Checklist, 98-99
Childbirth, 35
  birth of sibling, 33
Childhood or Adolescence - Differential Diagnosis, 11, 22, 27-30, 32-39, 45-46, 49, 91-124, 139
  acting-out behavior, 45-46
  Adjustment Disorder, 27-28, 39
  Anorexia Nervosa, 30, 33
  antisocial behavior, 27, 30, 36, 45-46, 94-99, 109, 117
  Antisocial Personality Disorder, 27
  Anxiety Disorders, 27-28, 30, 33, 36, 94-95

Childhood or Adolescence - Differential Diagnosis *(Continued)*
  Attention-Deficit Hyperactivity Disorder, 30, 32, 36
  Avoidant Disorder, 27
  Avoidant Personality Disorder, 27, 36
  Borderline Personality Disorder, 27
  Brief Reactive Psychosis, 27, 34
  Conduct Disorder, 27, 30, 32, 36, 45-46, 99
  Conversion Disorder, 37
  Defiant disorder (*see* Oppositional/Defiant Disorder)
  Depersonalization Disorder, 29
  depression, 29, 94-95, 99
  Disruptive Behavior Disorders, 27, 30, 32, 36, 45-46, 49, 99
  Dissociative Disorders, 22, 28-29, 37-38
  Dream Anxiety (Nightmare) Disorder, 29, 39, 109
  Dyssomnias, 29, 38
  Dysthymias, 36
  Eating Disorders, 30, 33, 95, 98-99
  Elective mutism, 30, 33
  Elimination Disorders, 30, 33, 97, 110
  Functional Encopresis, 30, 33
  Functional Enuresis, 30, 33, 97, 110
  Hyperactive disorder, (*see* Attention-Deficit Hyperactivity Disorder)
  Hypersomnia Disorder, 29
  Identity Disorder, 27
  incest, 11, 30, 103-104, 107, 112-114, 122, 138-139
  Insomnia Disorder, 29, 38
  Mood Disorders, 27, 29, 36, 94-95, 99
  Multiple Personality Disorder, 22, 28, 37, 103
  Obsessive-Compulsive Disorder, 28
  Oppositional Defiant Disorder, 32
  Organic Mental Disorders, 27

Childhood or Adolescence - Differential Diagnosis *(Continued)*
Panic Disorder, 22
Parasomnias, 29, 39
Personality Disorders, 22, 27-28, 36-38, 103
Psychoactive Substance Use Disorders, 27, 108-139
Psychogenic Amnesia, 29
psychological factors affecting physical condition, 27
Psychotic Disorders, 27, 34
PTSD, 28, 36, 105-112, 116-117
Schizophrenia, 27, 34
Schizophreniform Disorder, 27, 35
Separation Anxiety Disorder, 28, 30, 33, 36, 94-95, 111
sexual abuse, 91-100, 105-112, 116-117, 119-120
Sexual Disorders, 27
Simple phobia, 28
Sleep Disorders, 29, 38-39, 94-95, 97, 99, 106-110, 112
Sleep Terror Disorder, 29, 39, 107
Sleep-Wake Schedule Disorder, 29
Sleepwalking Disorder, 39
Somatization Disorder, 94, 111
Somatoform Disorder, 27, 37, 94, 111
Childhood sexual abuse, 22, 91-100, 105-112, 116-117, 119-120, 143-145
effects on adults, 100-105, 109-124
Children's Impact of Traumatic Events Scale, 117
Chowchilla school-bus kidnapping, 3-4, 106, 112
Chronic illness, 10, 39, 144
Chronic mood disorder - Dysthymia, 36, 67-68
Chronic pain syndromes, 22, 24
childhood physical/sexual trauma, 22
Chronic PTSD, 2, 15, 113, 139
Civic duties, 158

Civil suits, 137, 157
Civil War, The, 9, 85
Clinging behavior - child/adolescent, 94-96, 111
Coercive persuasion as stressor, 38, 108
Cognitive difficulties - SAV, 95, 101, 103, 105
Collateral reports, 18-19, 44, 71, 119-120, 141, 147-148, 151
Combat, 9-11, 31, 34, 38, 73-87, 114-115, 123-124, 142-144, 146-147
Civil War, The, 9, 85
Korean War, 74, 79, 146
Vietnam conflict, 9-10, 73-87, 115, 143-144, 146-147
World War I, 9, 74, 142
World War II, 9, 78-79, 83, 114, 146
Combat efficiency, 79, 81
Combat exhaustion, 10
Combat experiences, 78, 82, 115, 123-124, 160
acute reactions to, 82, 86
amount and severity of, 78, 123-124
Combat fatigue, 10, 74
Combat neurosis, 10
Combatants - Vietnam conflict, 79-80, 82
Commanding officers - Problems, 81-82, 139
Commercial product defects, 160
Communality/Community, loss of, 12, 17, 25, 143
Compensation claims, 15-17, 25-26, 74, 78, 83, 137-138, 144-146, 159-160
Compensation laws, 74, 85, 157, 159-160
Compensation neurosis, 74
Complaint filing - lawsuits, 171-172
Compounding disorders *(see Confounding factors/disorders)*
Compulsions *(see Obsessive-Compulsive Disorder)*
Compulsive personality *(see Obsessive-Compulsive Disorder)*
Concealment of abuse, 116, 118
Concentration camps, 11, 114

Concentration difficulties, 1, 63-64, 68, 70, 78, 94-95, 101, 103, 106, 108, 110, 112, 115
  adult SAV, 101, 103, 106, 110, 112, 115
  child/adolescent SAV, 94-95, 106, 108, 110
Concurrent disorders, 3, 16-17, 143-144
Concussion, 18, 24, 63, 69-71, 74
Conduct Disorder, 27, 30, 32, 36, 43, 45-46, 49, 99
Conduct problems - SAV, 94-96, 99, 101, 105, 108-109, 111-112, 117
Confidential communications, 177-183
Confidentiality questions, 172
Conflicting testimony, 85
Confounding factors/disorders, 14-17, 32-39, 40-49, 160
Confusion in reporting details of trauma, 70-71, 140
Conjugal relationships (*see* Marital problems)
Constriction of affect, 77, 106, 110, 140
Contradictory reports, 70-71, 85, 138, 140, 142, 146
Control, loss of, 77, 121
Conversion Disorder, 30, 37, 142-143
Conversion hysteria, 10
Cooperation, lack of, 15, 44-45, 47-48, 84
Coping mechanisms/resources, 77, 120, 140, 161
Corruption, Vietnam conflict, 81
Cowardice, 74
Criminal behavior - PTSD as defense, 85-87
Criminal prosecution, 158
Criminal suits, 137, 157
Cross-examination, 173, 175, 187-191
Cruelty to animals - child/adolescent, 45
Cultural influences, 79, 142-148
  Vietnam conflict, 79
Cumulative trauma (*see* Stressors, multiple)

Curiosity, sexual - child/adolescent SAV, 96, 98

Deafness, 34
Death of significant others, 11-12, 16, 30-31, 33-34, 37, 69, 77, 82, 107, 160
Defense attorney, roles of, 15-17, 23-24, 167-193
Defiant disorder (*see* Oppositional/Defiant Disorder)
Defining terms - report writing, 164-165
Delayed PTSD, 14-15, 113, 117, 138, 160
Delayed stress, 76
Delinquent peers - Association with and Conduct Disorder, 32
Delinquency (*see* Antisocial behavior; Antisocial Personality Disorder; Conduct Disorder)
  child/adolescent SAV, 96, 117
Delusional Disorder, 30, 34
Delusions, 68
Denial, 77, 140, 149
Denial, by professionals, 2-5, 91, 112, 139, 145-146, 148
Dependence - alcohol/caffeine, 42
Dependent Personality Disorder, 36-37
Depersonalization Disorder, 29-30, 38
Depositions, 169-170, 172, 187
Depression, 2, 26, 29, 35, 63, 67-69, 75-76, 78, 84, 94-95, 97, 99-101, 104-106, 111-115, 118-119, 123, 160
  adult SAV, 100-101, 104-105, 111, 113-115, 118-119, 123
  child/adolescent SAV, 94-95, 97, 99, 105-106, 111-112, 116
Derealization (*see* Depersonalization Disorder)
DEROs (*see* Tours of duty - Vietnam conflict)
Destruction of property - child/adolescent, 45
Detachment (*see* Psychic numbing)
Deterioration (*see* Post-trauma changes)

Deterioration of relationships (*see* Interpersonal problems)

Determination of extent of stressors, 12-13

Determination of qualifications - expert witnesses, 184

Developmental history, 74

Developmental problems, 13-14, 36, 82, 110, 144, 147, 163

Diagnostic errors, 78, 84, 118, 139, 148-151

Differential Diagnosis - Adults

  Adjustment Disorder, 26, 30, 39, 64-65, 73

  Antisocial Personality Disorder, 17, 30, 40-46, 48-49, 142, 150

  Anxiety Disorders, 28, 30, 36, 63, 64-67, 118, 160

  Avoidant Personality Disorder, 36

  Bipolar Disorder, 35, 67-68

  Borderline Personality Disorder, 22, 27, 30, 118

  Brief Reactive Psychosis, 27-28, 30, 34-35, 63, 86 .

  Conduct Disorder, 27, 30, 49

  Conversion Disorder, 30, 37, 142-143

  Delusional Disorder, 30, 34

  Dependent Personality Disorder, 36-37

  Depersonalization Disorder, 29-30, 38

  depression, 2, 26, 35, 63, 67-69, 75-76, 78, 84, 100-101, 104-105, 111, 113-115, 118-119, 123, 160

  Dissociative Disorders, 28-30, 37-38, 86, 103, 118

  Dream Anxiety (Nightmare) Disorder, 29-30, 39, 42, 63, 75

  Dyssomnias, 29-30, 38-39, 63-64, 68

  Dysthymia, 36, 67-68

  Generalized Anxiety Disorder, 63-65, 118, 160

  Hypersomnia, 29-30, 68

  Hypochondriasis, 30, 37

  incest, 11, 30, 107, 112-114, 122

Differential Diagnosis - Adults (*Continued*)

  insomnia, 29-30, 38, 63-64, 68

  malingering, 40, 43-46, 71, 74, 86, 149, 151

  Manic depression (*see* Bipolar Disorder)

  Mood Disorders, 2, 27, 29-30, 35-36, 63, 67-69, 75-76, 78, 84, 100-101, 104-105, 111, 113-115, 118-119, 123, 160

  Multiple Personality Disorder, 22, 28, 30, 37, 103

  Narcissistic Personality, 36

  Organic Mental Disorders, 26-27, 30, 42

  Panic Disorder, 22, 28, 36, 63-65, 67

  Paranoid Personality Disorder, 30

  Parasomnias, 29-30, 39, 42, 63, 75, 147

  Personality Disorders, 17, 22, 26-28, 30, 34-37, 40-48, 103, 118

  Psychoactive Substance Use Disorders, 27, 30, 40-42, 48-49, 63, 65, 79-81, 84, 101, 103-104, 117, 140, 142, 147, 150

  Psychogenic Fugue, 30, 38

  Psychotic Disorders, 27-28, 30, 34-35, 63, 68, 86, 139, 143

  PTSD, 1-4, 9-26, 28, 36, 40, 42-45, 50, 63-64, 70-71, 73-79, 82-87, 92, 105-124, 137-151, 157-165, 191

  Schizophrenia, 27, 30, 34-35, 139, 143

  Schizophreniform Disorder, 27, 30, 35

  Schizotypal Personality Disorder, 30, 34

  sexual abuse as children - long-term effects on adults, 100-105, 109-124

  Sleep Disorders, 29-30, 38-39, 42, 63-64, 68, 75, 147

  Sleep Terror Disorder, 29-30, 39, 147

Differential Diagnosis - Adults *(Continued)*
  Sleepwalking Disorder, 30, 39
  Somatoform Disorders, 27, 30, 37, 40-41, 46, 48-49, 142
  Somatoform Pain Disorders, 37, 142
Differential Diagnosis in Childhood or Adolescence *(see* Childhood or Adolescence - Differential Diagnosis)
Differential responses to duration of stress, 13
Diminished capacity, legal defense, 85-87
Direct courtroom examination, 173-188
Disability, 68, 75, 78, 83, 157, 160-164
  claims, 75, 83, 160
  estimation of, 157, 161-164
  ratings, 163-164
Disbelief, 75-76, 78
Discipline, harsh - children/adolescents, 32, 145
Discipline problems - Vietnam, 81
Disclosure - confidential communications, 177-183
Disclosure of facts - expert opinion, 184
Disclosure - reports/records, 164-165, 170-171
Disclosure of sexual abuse, 100, 118, 120-122
  concealment of sexual abuse, 116, 118
"Discovery" methods - Legal procedures for, 169-170, 172, 187
Discovery provisions - Legal determinations of fact, 164
Discrediting testimony, 188-191
Discrepancies in reporting *(see* Self-reports, confusion)
Disease in family member or other person as stressor, 37
Dishonesty - Vietnam conflict, 81
Dismemberment, 66-67, 159, 161-162

Disruptive Behavior Disorders, 27, 30, 32, 36, 43, 45-46, 49, 84, 97
  Attention-Deficit Hyperactivity Disorder, 30, 32, 36
  Conduct Disorder, 27, 30, 32, 36, 43, 45-46, 49, 99
  Oppositional/Defiant Disorder, 32
Dissociation, 85-86, 94-95, 101, 103, 107, 109, 112, 114, 140, 147
  adult SAV, 101, 103, 109, 114
  child/adolescent SAV, 94-95, 107, 109, 112
Dissociative Disorders, 28-30, 37-38, 86, 103, 118
  Depersonalization Disorder, 29-30, 38
  Hysterical Dissociative States, 86
  Multiple Personality Disorder, 22, 28, 30, 37, 103
  Psychogenic Amnesia, 29, 38, 69, 101, 103, 110, 114, 140, 147
  Psychogenic Fugue, 30, 38
Distress, level of, 44
Distrust, 14-15, 44-45, 64, 79-80, 114-115, 117, 120-121
  adult SAV, 114-115, 121
  child/adolescent SAV, 117, 120
Divorce, 10 *(see also* Marital problems)
Dizziness *(see* Vertigo)
Documentation - learned treatises, 185-186
Domestic battering, 103, 145
Dream Anxiety (Nightmare) Disorder, 1, 29-30, 39, 42, 63, 75
Drug abuse, 79-81, 103-104, 108, 138-140, 142, 147, 150
  adult SAV, 79-81, 103-104
  child/adolescent SAV, 108, 138-139
Dubiousness regarding diagnosis, 3-4, 91, 112, 139, 145-146, 148
Dyssomnias, 29-30, 38-39, 63-64, 68
  Hypersomnia Disorder, 29-30, 68

Dyssomnias *(Continued)*
  Insomnia Disorder, 29-30, 39,
    63-64, 68
  Sleep-Wake Schedule Disorder,
    29
Dysthymia, 36, 67-68

Early marriage, adolescent SAV,
  95, 98
Eating Disorders, 30, 33, 95, 98-99,
  101-102, 118
  Anorexia Nervosa, 30, 33
  child/adolescent SAV, 95, 98-99
  obesity, 101-102
ECT *(see* Electroconvulsive therapy)
Educational background, 23, 71
EEG *(see* Electroencephalogram)
Ego defenses, 77, 140, 161
Elective mutism, 30, 33
Electroconvulsive therapy, 35
Electroencephalogram, 71
Elimination Disorders, 30, 33, 97,
  110
  child/adolescent SAV, 97, 110
  Functional Encopresis, 30, 33
  Functional Enuresis, 30, 33
Emergency technicians, 25-26
Emigration, 34
Emotional lability, 18, 106, 111,
  121, 144
Emotional numbing *(see* Psychic
  numbing)
Employers' responsibilities, 159
Employment problems, 2, 124
Encopresis, 30, 33, 110
Enduring stressors, 2, 13, 15
Enuresis, 30, 33, 97, 110
Environmental complications *(see*
  Confounding factors/disor-
  ders)
Environmental support *(see* Support
  systems)
Estimating disability, 157, 161-164
Estrangement *(see* Psychic numbing)
Ethnic differences, 147-148
Evaluation *(see* Assessment; Collater-
  al reports; Psychological eval-
  uation; Self-evaluation
  SAV; Self-Evaluation of Diffi-
  culties Questionnaire)
Evaluation errors, 118, 148-151
Evaluation problems, 15, 146-149

Evaluations - Conflict of interests
  and, 145
Evasiveness, 140
Evidence, admissibility of, 184
Evidentiary Rules, 174-185
Exacerbation of condition, 21-22,
  161-162
Exaggerated PTSD, 137-151
Exaggeration of symptoms, 44-49, 71
Examination order - judicial, 179
Exclusion of witnesses, 177-178
Exclusionary Rules, 179-180
Exhaustion, 14 *(see also* Fatigue)
Exhibitionism - child/adolescent
  SAV, 96, 98
Expectedness of events *(see* Anticipa-
  tion of disaster)
Expert witness roles, 23-24, 158-
  159, 162-165, 167-193
Extent of stressors - determination,
  12-13
External incentives for symptoms are
  not present, 47-48
Extortion of SAV, 108
Extreme stressors *(see* Stressors; se-
  verity of)

Fabricated military experience, 86,
  144
Factitious Disorder, 40-41, 47-48,
  138
  Münchausen's syndrome, 138
Factitious grief, 144
Factitious symptoms of PTSD, 138,
  142-143, 151
Factual disclosures - legal witnesses,
  184
Failure to comply *(see* Noncompli-
  ance with psychological e-
  valuation)
Faintness *(see* Vertigo)
Faking, 43, 46, 50, 149-151
Familial patterns, 46, 49, 68
Family history of high incidents of dis-
  orders, 49
Family relationships, 78, 120, 124,
  144, 160
  stability, 78, 124, 144, 160
Fantasy - confusion, 140, 144
Fathers, incestuous, 103-104, 138-
  139

Fatigue, 14, 29, 39, 63-64, 68, 70
  child/adolescent, 29, 39
Fear of men - SAV, 101-102, 109,
  114
Fears, 17, 64, 66, 94-96, 99, 108-
  109, 139-140, 144, 148
Federal Rules of Evidence, 174-185
Fees, expert witness, 169
Fifth Amendment privilege, 180
Fighting - child/adolescent, 45, 94-
  95, 97
Financial problems, 13, 16, 68
Firesetting - child/adolescent, 45
Flashbacks, 63, 68, 85, 95, 101-102,
  107-109, 118, 147
  adult SAV, 101-102, 109, 118
  child/adolescent SAV, 95, 107-
    109
Follow-up evaluation, 124
Forensic issues, 157-166
Forensic procedures and guidelines,
  167-193
Foundation for testimony - expert
  witness, 186
Fugue (see Psychogenic Fugue)
Functional Encopresis, 30, 33, 110
Functional Enuresis, 30, 33, 97, 110

GAF Scale (see Global Assessment of
  Functioning Scale)
Generalized Anxiety Disorder, 63-
  65, 118, 160
Generational conflict - Vietnam, 79
Genital exposure (see Exhibitionism -
  child/adolescent SAV)
Giddiness (see Vertigo)
Global Assessment of Functioning
  Scale, 12
Grief, 30-31, 40, 69, 144
  factitious, 144
Gross stress reaction, 10, 73
Group therapy - SAV, 122
Guilt, 1, 15, 43-44, 68, 94-95, 97,
  99, 101-102, 106, 108, 111-
  112, 117, 121-122
  adult SAV, 101-102, 111, 115
  child/adolescent SAV, 94-95, 97,
    99, 106, 108, 111-112,
    117, 121-122

Hallucinations, 68, 76, 108, 148
Head injury, 11, 24, 63, 69-71, 74
  concussion, 18, 24, 63, 69-71,
    74
Headaches, 18, 70, 95, 101-102,
  106, 111-112, 115
Helplessness, feelings of, 83, 107,
  117, 122
Historical summary of PTSD, 9-10,
  73-74
History of client's functioning, 23,
  43, 71, 120 (see also Military
  history of patient)
Histrionic Personality Disorder, 30,
  36-37, 48, 140, 142
Holocaust, victims of, 138, 145
Hospitalism, 41, 47-49
  Factitious Disorder, 40-41, 47-
    48, 138
  Somatization Disorder, 40-41,
    46, 48-49, 94, 111, 142
Hospitalization, 33, 47, 49, 104,
  144, 179
  legal proceedings for, 179
  young age, 33
Hostage-taking - Vietnam veterans,
  85
Hostility (see Anger)
Hyperactive disorder (see Attention-
  Deficit Hyperactivity Disor-
  der)
Hyperalertness (see Hypervigilance)
Hyperparathyroidism, 41
Hypersomnia, 29-30, 68
Hyperthyroidism, 65
Hypervigilance, 64, 108, 110, 115
Hypochondriasis, 30, 37
Hypoglycemia, 65
Hypomanic disorder (see Bipolar Dis-
  order)
Hypothetical questions of expert
  witnesses, 185-186
Hysteria, 147
Hysterical Dissociative States, 86
Hysterical personality (see Histrionic
  Personality Disorder)
Hysterical psychosis (see Brief Reac-
  tive Psychosis; Factitious Dis-
  order)

Idealistic illusions (see Invulnerability, loss of)

Identity confusion, 75, 137, 143-144, 151
Identity Disorder, 27, 103
Idiosyncratic responses, 14, 141
Illness, 10, 13, 36, 39, 47-49, 68, 139-140, 144, 163
Illusions - SAV, 109
Imagined PTSD, 137-151
Immigration, 33-34
Impulsive behavior, 17, 94, 96, 106, 111-112, 115
   adult SAV, 106, 115
   child/adolescent SAV, 94, 96, 106, 111-112
Inability to discuss losses, 40, 140
Incentives for production of symptoms are not present, 47-48
Incest, 11, 30, 103-104, 107, 112-114, 122, 138-139
Incestuous fathers, 103-104, 138-139
Inconsistent symptoms, 44, 142
Increased stress (see Life events)
Indirect exposure to trauma, 25-26, 37
Injury, 11, 13, 18, 24-25, 29, 137, 139-140, 159, 163
Insanity, legal defense, 85-86
Insomnia Disorder, 29-30, 38-39, 63-64, 68
Institutionalization, 32
Insurance coverage, 159-160
Interpersonal problems, 1, 10, 13, 17-18, 36, 38, 41, 43, 48, 63, 68, 82, 94-95, 101-103, 110, 112-114, 116, 123, 142, 163
   adult SAV, 94-95, 101-103, 110, 112-113, 116, 123
   child/adolescent SAV, 94-95, 97, 110, 114, 116
   commanding officers, 82
   marital problems, 1, 10, 13, 17, 38, 41, 68, 102-103
   military, 82, 142
   other, 13, 17, 43, 48, 63
Interrogation - Order and presentation of, 175-176
Interviewing techniques, 14-15, 18, 44, 71, 79, 85-86, 116-120, 139-141, 147-149, 151

Interviews with others, 18-19, 44, 71, 119, 141, 147-148, 151
Introduction of expert witnesses, 177
Intrusive thoughts - SAV, 103, 107, 114, 117, 121-123
Invasion of privacy (see Privacy)
Involuntary symptoms, 142-143 (see also Somatoform Disorders)
Invulnerability, loss of, 14, 77
Irritability, 17, 70, 94, 108, 110
   adult SAV, 110
   child/adolescent SAV, 94, 108, 110
Isolation (see Withdrawal)

Jackson Structured Interview, 118-119
Jargon, use of, 165
Jitteriness (see Autonomic lability)
Job loss, 10, 160
Juries, roles of, 192-193

Kidnapping, 3-4, 12, 106, 112
Korean War, 74, 79, 146

Labile personality (see Bipolar Disorder)
Lack of cooperation, 15, 44-45, 47-48
Lack of trust (see Distrust)
Language or speech disorders, 33
"Last straw" phenomenon, 162
Latent conditions (see Predisposing factors; Predisposition; Pre-existing conditions/vulnerabilities)
Law of Torts, 21, 157-159, 161-162, 164
Lawsuits, 1-3, 137, 157-159, 167-193
Lay witness opinions, 18-19, 44, 71, 119, 141, 147-148, 151, 183
Leadership, military, 80-81, 83
Leading questions - legal proceedings, 175-176
Learned treatises - expert witnesses, 185-186
Learning difficulties (see Academic problems - child/adolescent SAV)

Legal defense - PTSD used as, 85-87
Legal issues, 157-166
Legal obligations of citizens, 158-
    159
Legal problems - patient history of,
    13, 43
Level of distress (see Distress, level
    of)
Life events, 1, 10-13, 16-18, 23-24,
    31, 33-35, 37-38, 41, 68,
    75, 77-78, 82-83, 107, 157,
    160-164
    academic problems, 16, 94, 96,
        99, 108
    aging, 16, 38, 41, 49
    childbirth, 35
        birth of sibling, 33
    death of significant others, 11-
        12, 16, 30-31, 33-34,
        37, 69, 77, 82, 107, 160
    family problems, 16
    financial problems, 13, 16, 68
    job loss, 10, 160
    living circumstances, 13
    marital problems, 1, 10, 13, 17,
        38, 41, 68, 160
    medical disabilities, 16, 68, 75,
        78, 83, 157, 160-164
    parental loss, 16
    premorbid personality, 16, 18,
        23-24, 143-144, 161-
        162
    retirement, 16
    work disability, 68
Lifestyle alterations, 17
Litigation, 1-3, 12-13, 15-18, 22-24,
        43-44, 46, 49, 71, 137, 157-
        193
    court proceedings, 167-193
    patient's history of, 13, 43
    personal injury, 159-164
Loss, 14, 40, 75-76, 160, 162-164
    of communality/community, 12,
        17, 25, 143
    of control, 77, 121
    of function, 16, 162-164
    of invulnerability, 14, 77
    of meaning, 14, 81
    of predictability, 75-76
    of self-esteem/self-image, 14, 68,
        77, 94-95, 97, 101-102,
        104, 111, 122-123, 142

Louisville Behavior Checklist, 97
Lupus (see Systemic lupus erythema-
    tosus)
Lying, 45, 142, 150
    child/adolescent, 45

Major affective disorders (see
    Mood Disorders)
Major Depression (see Depression)
Malicious persecution (see Persecu-
    tion)
Malingered PTSD, 137-156
Malingering, 40, 43-46, 71, 74, 86,
    137-151
Malnutrition, 11, 18, 24, 141
Manic-depression (see Bipolar Disor-
    der)
Marital history, 23
Marital problems, 1, 10, 13, 17, 38,
    41, 68, 103, 160
Masturbation, excessive - child/ado-
    lescent SAV, 96, 98, 108,
    112
Maternal deprivation (see Parenting
    problems, rejection)
Meaning, loss of, 14, 81
Meaning of stressors, 13-14, 81-82,
    137, 140-141, 143-144
Media coverage of PTSD, 3, 85, 87,
    138
Medical disabilities, 16, 68, 159-164
Medical evacuation - Vietnam, 76,
    79
Medical evaluation, 18, 40-42, 47-
    49, 69-71, 162-164
Medical expenses, 159
Medical history, 13, 23, 40, 47-49,
    71
Medication use/abuse, 47-48
Memories, intrusive, 75, 103, 107,
    114, 117, 121-123
Memory problems, 63, 106
Mental disorders - concurrent, 3, 16-
    17, 143-144
Mental health professionals - expert
    witness functions, 157-193
Mental retardation, 33, 36
Mental status, 119, 141
Migraine headaches (see Head-
    aches)

Military combat, 9-11, 29, 38, 73-
    87, 114-115, 123-124, 142-
    144, 146-147
  Civil War, The, 9, 85
  Korean War, 74, 79, 146
  Vietnam conflict, 9-10, 73-87,
    115, 143-144, 146-147
  World War I, 9, 74, 142
  World War II, 9, 78-79, 82, 114,
    146
Military efficiency, 79, 81
Military history of patient, 23, 71,
    86, 138-141, 143-144
Military leadership, 80-81, 83
Military morale, 80-82
Minimization of symptoms, 44, 140
Minnesota Multiphasic Personality
    Inventory, 46, 50, 119, 149-
    151
Misdiagnosis, 78, 84, 118, 139, 148-
    151
  Vietnam veterans, 78, 84, 139
Mitigation of punishment, 85
MMPI (see Minnesota Multiphasic
    Personality Inventory)
Monetary claims, 142
Monetary gains, 43, 46, 49
Mood Disorders, 2, 27, 29-30, 35-
    36, 63, 67-69, 75-76, 78,
    84, 100, 118
  Bipolar Disorder, 35, 67-68
  Depression, 2, 29, 35, 63, 67-
    69, 75-76, 78, 84, 100, 118
  Dysthymia, 36, 67-68
Morale, military, 80-82
Motor agitation/retardation, 68
Mourning (see Grief)
Multiple Personality Disorder, 22,
    28, 30, 37, 103
Multiple physical symptoms, 40-41,
    47-49
Multiple sclerosis, 41
Multiple stressors, 2, 12, 14, 21-26,
    39, 107, 143, 151
Multiple surgeries, 41, 47-48
Münchausen's syndrome, 138 (see
    also Factitious Disorder)
Muscle tension, 64

Nail biting - child/adolescent SAV,
    94-95, 111
Narcissism, 143-144

Narcissistic Personality Disorder, 36
Natural disasters, 38-39, 73, 76,
    145, 160
Negligence, 25-26, 44, 106, 158-
    159
Nervousness (see Anxiety)
Neurasthenia (see Dysthymia)
Neuropsychological evaluation, 18,
    71
Night terrors, 147
Nightmare disorder (see Dream Anxi-
    ety [Nightmare] Disorder)
Nightmares, 1, 29, 39, 42, 63, 68,
    75, 94-96, 101-102, 109,
    115, 139, 146-148
  child/adolescent SAV, 94-97,
    107, 109
Noncompliance with psychological
    evaluation, 15, 44-45, 47-48
Numbing (see Psychic numbing)
Numerous stressors (see Stressors,
    multiple)

Obesity - adult SAV, 101-102
Obsessive-Compulsive Disorder, 28
  ruminations, 64, 75
Occupational difficulties, 10, 13,
    150
Occupational disability, 159
Occupational history, 23, 71
Operational fatigue, 10
Opinion, bases for expert, 183, 185-
    186
Opposing counsel, style of, 187-188
Oppositional behavior, 97, 110
Oppositional/Defiant Disorder, 32
Optic symptoms, 70
Organic brain syndromes, 18, 24,
    63, 69-71, 74
  malnutrition, 11, 18, 24, 141
  concussion, 18, 24, 63, 69-71,
    74
Organic disease, 37, 41
Organic mental disorders, 26-27, 30,
    42
Orgasmic difficulties - SAV, 102, 104
Over-reactive affect, 71, 148

Pain medication (see Medication
    use/abuse)
Palpitations (see Autonomic lability)
Panic Disorder, 22, 28, 36, 63-67

Paranoid disorder (*see* Delusional Disorder)

Paranoid Personality Disorder, 30

Parasomnias, 29-30, 39, 42, 63, 68, 75, 107, 147

    Dream Anxiety (Nightmare) Disorder, 29-30, 39, 42, 63, 68, 75

    Sleep Terror Disorder, 29-30, 39, 107, 147

    Sleepwalking Disorder, 30, 39

Parenting problems, 32-33, 101-104, 107, 138-139, 144

    absence, 32, 144

    abuse, 103-104, 138-139

    alcohol abuse, 32

    incestuous fathers, 103-104, 138-139

    overprotection, 33

    rejection, 32, 107

    of SAV, 101-103

Parents/relatives of victims, 11

Passivity, 122

Patient history, 13, 23, 43, 71, 120, 141, 151 (*see also* Military history of patient)

Patient role, need to be in, 41, 47, 137-138, 142-143

Patient-therapist privilege, 178-183

Peers of Vietnam veterans, 85-86, 144

Persecution, 39, 145, 158

Personal injury litigation, 159-164

Personality Disorders, 17, 26-28, 30, 34-37, 40-49, 68, 139-140, 142-144, 148, 150-151

    Antisocial, 17, 27, 30, 40-49, 142, 150

    Avoidant, 27, 36

    Borderline, 22, 27, 30, 118

    Dependent, 36-37

    Dysthymia, 36, 67-68

    Histrionic, 30, 36-37, 48, 140, 142

    Multiple, 22, 28, 30, 37, 103

    Narcissistic, 36

    Paranoid, 30

    Schizoid, 140

    Schizotypal, 30, 34

Pessimism - child/adolescent SAV, 94

Pets, loss of, 33

Phobic avoidance (*see* Avoidance behavior)

Phobic behavior - child/adolescent, 28, 94-95, 99, 101-102, 105, 110, 119

Photocopied records, 170-171

Physical complaints, 40-41, 48

    unexplained, 38, 49

Physical damage suits, 158-160

Physical disorders/disease, 35, 37, 40-41, 47-49, 65

    exposure to people with, 37

Physical effects of sexual abuse, 94-95, 97-98, 101-102

Physical fatigue (*see* Fatigue)

Physical illness, 10, 13, 36, 39, 47-49, 68, 139-140, 144, 163

Physical injury, 11, 13, 18, 24-25, 29, 137, 139-140, 159, 163

    concussion, 18, 24, 63, 69-71, 74

    head injury, 11, 24, 63, 69-71, 74

Physical problems - SAV, 94-95, 97-98, 101-102, 105-106, 111-112, 115-116

Physical symptoms, multiple/vague, 40-41, 47-49

Physical trauma (*see* Physical injury)

Physical violence, 12, 145

Physicians' estimate of physical disability, 162

Playing behavior - child SAV, 106, 109, 112, 120

Pornography shows - child/adolescent SAV, 107

Porphyria, 41

Post-concussion syndrome (*see* Concussion)

Post-trauma changes, 12-13, 16, 23, 160, 162-164

Post-traumatic play - SAV, 120

Post-Traumatic Stress Disorder, 1-4, 9-26, 28, 36, 40, 42-45, 50, 63-64, 68, 70-71, 73-79, 82-87, 92, 105-124, 137-151, 157-165, 191

    affect, restriction of, 77, 106, 110, 140

    aggressivity, 17, 43, 97, 99, 109

Post-Traumatic Stress Disorder *(Continued)*

anger, 17, 43, 78, 83, 94-95, 97, 99, 105, 110, 112, 114, 121-122, 150

anxiety, 26, 46, 70, 75-76, 94-95, 97, 101-102, 104-107, 111-113, 115-116, 118-119, 146, 150

autonomic arousal, 64, 68, 75, 77-78, 108, 110-112, 118, 137, 139, 149

autonomic lability, 18

children and adolescents, 28, 36, 105-112, 116-117

chronic states, 2, 15, 113, 139

delayed reactions, 14-15, 113, 117, 138, 160

depression, 94-95, 97, 99-101, 104-106, 111-116, 118-119, 123

diagnostic criteria, 108-116

distrust, 14-15, 44-45, 64, 79-80, 114-115, 117, 120-121

emotional lability, 18, 106, 111, 121, 144

guilt, 1, 15, 43-44, 68, 94-95, 97, 99, 101-102, 106, 108, 111-112, 117, 121-122

headaches, 18, 70, 95, 101-102, 106, 111-112, 115

historical summary, 9-10, 73-74

impulsive behavior, 17, 94, 96, 106, 111-112, 115

interviewing techniques, 14-15, 18, 44, 71, 79, 85-86, 116-120, 139-141, 147-149, 151

irritability, 17, 70, 94, 108, 110

psychic numbing, 40, 42-43, 45, 75, 77, 109-110, 112, 114-115, 119, 121-122

stressors, 10-13
  evaluation of, 10-26, 75-77
  meaning of, 13-14, 81-82, 137, 140-141, 143
  multiple, 2, 12, 14, 21-26, 39, 107, 143, 151
  severity of, 2, 10-26

Post-Traumatic Stress Disorder diagnosed as
  battle fatigue, 74
  battle stress, 10
  combat exhaustion, 10
  combat fatigue, 10, 74
  combat neurosis, 10
  conversion hysteria, 10
  gross stress reactions, 10, 73
  operational fatigue, 10
  railway spine, 74
  rape trauma syndrome, 10
  shell shock, 74
  traumatic neurosis, 10, 113, 146, 159
  traumatic war neurosis, 10

Post-war adjustment - complications of Vietnam veterans, 73-86

Predictability (see Loss, of predictability)

Predisposing factors, 13, 19-24, 28, 32-39, 47-49

Predisposition, 19-24, 36, 74, 78-79, 86, 157, 161-162

Pre-existing conditions/vulnerabilities, 16-24, 26, 28, 32-39, 47-49, 143-144, 161-162

Pregnancy - adolescent SAV, 95, 98

Prejudiced evaluations, 145, 148, 151

Prejudices in war, 81

Premorbid personality, 16, 18, 23-24, 35-36, 120, 143-144, 161-162

Preparation of witness, 187-193

Preparedness (see Anticipation of disaster)

Pretrial discovery, 169-170, 172, 187

Primary Hypersomnia, 30 (see *also* Hypersomnia)

Primary Insomnia, 30 (see *also* Insomnia Disorder)

Prior statements made by expert witnesses, 176-177

Privacy, 158, 165

Privilege waivers, 182

Privileged communication, 172, 177-183

Product liability laws, 157-159

Professional jargon, use of, 165

Prognosis, 15-17, 120
Projective techniques, 119, 149
Promiscuity - SAV, 96, 101, 104, 111
Prostitution - SAV, 96, 101, 104
Protection from disclosure - legal opinion and, 165
Proximate cause, 157, 160-161
Pseudologia fantastica, 144
Psychic loss, 14
Psychic numbing, 40, 42-43, 45, 75, 77, 109-110, 112, 114-115, 119, 121-122
Psychoactive Substance Use Disorders, 27, 30, 40-42, 48-49, 63, 65, 79-81, 84, 101, 103-104, 108, 117, 139-140, 142, 147, 150
  adult SAV, 101, 103-104, 117
  child/adolescent SAV, 27, 108, 139
Psychoanalytic influences, 74, 78-79, 86, 91
Psychogenic Amnesia, 29, 38, 69, 101, 103, 110, 114, 140, 147
Psychogenic Fugue, 30, 38
Psychogenic symptoms, 71
Psychological evaluation, 3, 12-30, 32-51, 69, 71, 74, 78-79, 81, 86, 97-99, 116-120, 124, 137-141, 143-145, 147-151, 157, 160-164, 190, 197-215
  bereavement as complication, 30-31, 40, 69
  Brecksville PTSD Inventory, 118
  Child Behavior Checklist, 98-99
  Children's Impact of Traumatic Events Scale, 117
  concurrent disorders, 3, 16-17, 143-144
  confounding factors/disorders, 14-17, 32-49, 160
  diagnostic interview, 71
  disability, 157, 160-164
  extent of stressors, 12-13
  follow-up, 124
  Global Assessment of Functioning Scale, 12

Psychological evaluation *(Continued)*
  grief as complication, 30-31, 40, 69
  interviews with others, 18-19, 44, 71, 119, 141, 147-148, 151
  Jackson Structured Interview, 118-119
  meaning of stressors, 13-14, 81-82, 137, 140-141, 143
  military history of patient, 23, 71, 86, 138-141, 144
  Minnesota Multiphasic Personality Inventory, 46, 50, 119, 149-151
  multiple stressors, 2, 12, 14, 21-26, 39, 107, 143, 151
  noncompliance with, 15, 44-45
  other symptoms, 17-19
  patient history, 13, 23, 43, 71, 120, 141, 151 (*see also* Military history of patient)
  physical injuries, 24-25, 162-164
  predisposing factors, 13, 19-24, 28, 32-39, 47-49
  predisposition, 19-24, 36, 74, 78-79, 86, 157, 161-162
  pre-existing conditions/vulnerabilities, 16-24, 26, 28, 32-39, 47-49, 143-144, 161-162
  premorbid personality, 16, 23-24, 35-36, 120, 143-144, 161-162
  problems in, 145-147
  Self-Evaluation of Difficulties Questionnaire, 50-51, 197-215
  Severity of Psychosocial Stressors Scale, 12
  sexual abuse, 91-124
  State-Trait Anxiety Inventory, 119
  stress-related diagnoses, 26-30
  Structured Clinical Interview for *DSM-III*, 118
  testing, 12, 46, 50, 97-99, 117-119, 149-151, 190
  variations in reactions, 19-24

Psychological factors affecting physical condition, 27, 30
Psychological history (see Psychological evaluation; Patient history)
Psychological meaning of stressors (see Stressors, meaning of)
Psychometric testing (see Testing)
Psychopathic Personality (see Antisocial Personality Disorder)
Psychopathology - SAV, 98-100
Psychosocial stress, 13, 29, 33-38
Psychotherapist-patient privilege, 178-183
Psychotic Disorders, 27-28, 30, 34-35, 63, 86, 139, 143
    Brief Reactive Psychosis, 27, 30, 34-35, 63, 68, 86
    child/adolescent, 27, 34
    Delusional Disorder, 30, 34
    Organic Mental Disorders, 26-27, 30, 42
    Schizophrenia, 27, 30, 34-35, 139, 143
    Schizophreniform Disorder, 27, 30, 35
Publicity (see Media coverage of PTSD)
Punishment, mitigation of, 85
Purdue Self-Concept Scale, 97

Qualifications as expert witness, 167, 184, 186, 188
Quarreling and fighting - child/adolescent, 45, 94-95, 97
Questioning victims, 14-15, 116-120, 139-140, 147-149
Questions, hypothetical - expert witnesses, 185-186
Questions, leading - Legal proceedings, 175-176

Railway spine, 74
Rape, 11, 19, 73, 75, 103, 138, 145, 160
    adolescent perpetrator, 45
    incest, 11, 30, 107, 112-114, 122
Rape trauma syndrome, 10
Recall of events, 1, 138, 140, 142

Records, photocopies of, 170-171
Records, release of, 165
Recovery (see Prognosis)
Recurrent associations (see Associations to event)
Recurrent stressors (see Stressors, multiple)
Re-experiencing of traumatic event, 1, 14, 45, 75-76, 106-109, 114-115, 119, 143
Refusal to comply (see Noncompliance with psychological evaluation)
Reintegration, 75-76
Relationship problems (see Interpersonal problems)
Relatives with high incidence of disorders, 49
Relevancy of information presented by expert witnesses, 184
Relinquishment of records, 165
Repeated victimization, 23, 103
Repetitive play - child/adolescent SAV, 106, 109
Repetitive thoughts - SAV, 101, 121
Report writing, 157-158, 164-165, 172
Reports by expert witnesses, 187
Repression, 121, 138-139
Rescuers, 25-26
Research regarding stressors, 10-12
Resentment, Vietnam conflict, 79, 81-84
Residence changes, frequent, 31
Residual PTSD (see Delayed PTSD)
Resisting discussion of trauma, 14-15, 40, 140
Responsiveness, diminished - SAV, 106-107
Restlessness, 63-64
Restriction of affect, 77, 106, 110, 140
Retaliation fears in SAV, 108
Retardation (see Mental retardation)
Rorschach imagery, 149
Rules of Evidence, 174-185
Ruminations, 64, 75
Running away from home - child/adolescent, 45, 96, 98-99, 111, 117

Schizoid Personality Disorder, 140

Schizophrenia, 27, 30, 34-35, 139, 143

Schizophreniform Disorder, 27, 30, 35

Schizotypal Personality Disorder, 30, 34

School dropout - child/adolescent, 98 (see also Running away from home - child/adolescent)

School history, 23, 71

School problems - child/adolescent SAV, 94-96, 99, 108

SCID (see Structured Clinical Interview for *DSM-III*)

Secondary conflicts, 150

Secondary gain, 43, 46, 49, 71, 74, 142, 144, 151, 160

not present or explainable, 47-48

Secondary stress, 14-17, 139, 143 (see also Life events)

Self-assessment by SAV, 105, 119, 121-122

Self-blame, 1, 121-122, 138

Self-defeating thoughts and behavior - SAV, 122-123

Self-destructive desire or behavior - SAV, 94, 100, 102, 104-105, 111, 118

child/adolescent SAV, 94, 111

Self-esteem/self-image loss, 14, 68, 77, 94-95, 97, 101-102, 104, 111, 122-123, 143

adult SAV, 101-102, 104, 111, 122-123

child/adolescent SAV, 94-95, 97, 111, 123

Self-evaluation - SAV, 105, 119, 121-122 (see also page 141)

Self-Evaluation of Difficulties Questionnaire, 50-51, 197-215

"Self-medication" - Alcohol abuse, 42

Self-reliance, loss of, 65

Self-reports,confusion, 44, 46-48, 138, 140

Separation Anxiety Disorder, 28, 30, 33, 36, 94-95, 111

Severity of Psychosocial Stressors Scale, 12

Severity of stressors, 2, 10-26

Sex rings - child/adolescent SAV, 107-108

Sexual abuse, 11, 91-124

adults, 100-105, 109-124

child/adolescent, 91-100, 105-112, 116-117, 119-120

clinical studies, 94-96

duration of, 93, 130, 135

empirical studies, 96-100

frequency of, 92, 120, 124

initial effects of, 93-100

long-term effects of, 100-105

research - methodological problems, 92-93

Sexual Abuse Trauma Syndrome, 92, 122

Sexual assault, 11, 23, 91-124

history of victim, 23

Sexual curiosity - child/adolescent SAV, 96, 98

Sexual delinquency - child-adolescent SAV, 45, 96

Sexual disorders, 27, 63

Sexual history of victim, 23

Sexual problems - SAV, 96, 98, 102, 104-105, 108-109, 112-114, 116, 118, 123 (see also page 163)

Shakiness (see Autonomic lability)

Sham PTSD, 149

Shame - child/adolescent SAV, 94-95, 97, 99

Shell-shock syndrome, 74

Signature, depositions, 170

Significant others - interviews with, 18-19, 71, 119, 141, 147-148, 151

Simple phobia, 28

Simulated PTSD, 142

Skepticism (see Denial)

Skin disorders - SAV, 100, 102

Slander, 158

Sleep difficulties, 29, 94-95, 97, 99, 101-102, 105-110, 112, 115, 137, 146

adult SAV, 101-102, 105, 109-110, 112, 115

child/adolescent SAV, 94-95, 97, 99, 106-110, 112

Sleep Disorders, 1, 29-30, 38-39, 42, 63-64, 68, 75, 107, 147

Sleep Disorders *(Continued)*
  Dyssomnias, 29-30, 38-39, 63-64, 68
    Hypersomnia Disorder, 29-30, 68
    Insomnia Disorder, 29-30, 38-39, 63-64, 68
    Sleep-Wake Schedule Disorder, 29
  Parasomnias, 1, 29-30, 39, 42, 68, 75, 107, 147
    Dream Anxiety (Nightmare) Disorder, 1, 29-30, 39, 42, 63, 68, 75
    Sleep Terror Disorder, 29-30, 39, 107, 147
    Sleepwalking Disorder, 30, 39
Sleep Terror Disorder, 29-30, 39, 107, 147
Sleep-Wake Schedule Disorder, 29
Sleepwalking Disorder, 30, 39
Social difficulties - SAV, 94-96, 98, 101-103, 105, 110, 116-117, 123
Social history, 23, 43
Social phobia, 28
Social support, 17, 25, 36, 44, 120-124
Social withdrawal (*see* Withdrawal)
Sociopathic personality (*see* Antisocial Personality Disorder)
Somatic complaints, 66, 94-95, 97, 101-102, 106, 111-112, 115-116
  adult SAV, 101-102, 111, 115
  child/adolescent SAV, 94-95, 97, 106, 111-112, 116
Somatization Disorder, 40-41, 46, 48-49, 94, 111, 142
  adult SAV, 111
  child/adolescent SAV, 94, 111
Somatoform Disorders, 27, 30, 37, 40-41, 46, 48-49, 142
  Conversion Disorder, 30, 37, 142-143
  Hypochondriasis, 30, 37
  Somatization Disorder, 40-41, 46, 48-49, 94, 111, 142
  Somatoform Pain Disorder, 37, 142
Somatoform Pain Disorder, 37, 142

Speech or language disorders, 33
Spousal abuse - SAV, 103, 145
STAI (*see* State-Trait Anxiety Inventory)
Startle reaction, 1, 63-64, 68, 108, 111, 119
Starvation, 141 (*see also* Malnutrition)
State-Trait Anxiety Inventory, 119
Stealing - child/adolescent, 45, 111
Stigmatization - sexual abuse, 117
Stomach ailments, 95, 101-102, 106, 111-112, 115
  adult SAV, 101-102, 111, 115
  child/adolescent SAV, 95, 106, 111-112
Stress disorders and crime, 86
Stress-related diagnoses, 26-30
Stressors, 10-13
  evaluation of, 10-26, 75
  existence of, 14, 86, 139-141, 150
  meaning of, 13-14, 81-82, 137, 140-141, 143
  multiple, 2, 12-14, 21-26, 34, 36, 39, 107, 143, 151
  severity of, 2, 10-26
Structured Clinical Interview for *DSM-III*, 118
Structured interviews, 141, 151
Subpoenas, 165, 167-172
Substance abuse - child/adolescent SAV, 96
Substance use disorders (*see* Psychoactive Substance Use Disorders)
Suggestibility/patient, 47
Suicidal ideation, 64, 68, 94-95, 100, 104, 111, 114-115
  adult SAV, 64, 68, 100, 104, 111, 114-115
  child/adolescent SAV, 94-95, 111
Suicide attempts - SAV, 105
Suits (*see* Lawsuits)
Summons, lawsuits, 171-172
Support systems, 17, 25, 36, 44, 120-124
Suppression, 76-77
Surgeries, multiple, 41, 47-48
Survival attitudes, 81, 114, 141
Survivor theory, 115

Suspiciousness, 43 (*see also* Distrust)
Symbolic meaning, 14, 109
Symptoms, no incentives present, 47-48
Systemic lupus erythematosus, 41

Tantrums - child/adolescent SAV, 94-95, 110
Testimony, foundation - expert witnesses, 186
Testing, 12, 46, 50, 97-99, 117-119, 149-151, 190
    Brecksville PTSD Inventory, 118
    Child Behavior Checklist, 98-99
    Children's Impact of Traumatic Events Scale, 117
    Global Assessment of Functioning Scale, 12
    Jackson Structured Interview, 118-119
    legal challenge of, 190
    Louisville Behavior Checklist, 97
    Minnesota Multiphasic Personality Inventory, 46, 50, 119, 149-151
    projective techniques, 119, 149
    Purdue Self-Concept Scale, 97
    Rorschach, 149
    Severity of Psychosocial Stressors Scale, 12
    State-Trait Anxiety Inventory, 119
    Structured Clinical Interview for *DSM-III*, 118
Therapeutic understanding and goals, 75-76, 79, 85-86, 120-123
Therapist as expert witness, 167-193
Therapist-patient privilege, 178-183
Thin Skull Principle, 21-22, 161-162
Thoughts, problems with, 64, 75, 101-103, 107, 114, 117, 121-123
    intrusive, 75, 103, 107, 114, 117, 121-123
    repetitive, 101, 121
    ruminative, 64, 75
    self-defeating, 122-123
Threats of harm to self or others as stressors, 11, 25, 38
Thyroid disorders, 65
Time distortion, 140

Toilet training, 33
Tort law, 21, 157-159, 161-162, 164
Tours of duty - Vietnam conflict, 80-81
Traumatic neurosis, 10, 113, 146, 159
Traumatic war neurosis, 10
Treatises (*see* Learned treatises - expert witnesses)
Treatment needs of victims - evaluation of, 163
Trials - Order of proceedings, 172-174
Truancy - child/adolescent SAV, 96, 98, 111

Unbidden images (*see* Memories, intrusive)
Uncomplicated bereavement, 30-31, 40
Uncooperative behavior, 15, 44-45, 47-48, 84
Unemployment, 10, 160
Unexpectedness of trauma, 22-23, 81, 160
Unpredictable behavior (*see* Impulsive behavior)
Unreality, 138
Unresolved grief, 31, 40

Vague physical symptoms, 40-41, 47-49
Venereal disease - child/adolescent SAV, 94
Vertigo, 18, 66, 106, 111
Veterans, peers of, 85-86, 144
Veterans Administration, problems with, 83-84, 139, 142, 145
Victim compensation, 146, 158-159
Victimization - sexual assault, 23, 102-103, 121
Vietnam conflict, 3, 9-10, 73-89, 138, 143-144, 147
    and publicity, 3, 85, 87, 138
    and research, 9-10
Vietnam veterans, 3, 10, 73-89, 115, 120, 138-140, 143-147
Violent crimes - Vietnam veterans, 85-87, 141, 145
Vocational background, 23

Voluntary symptoms, 40, 142-143
  (*see also* Factitious Disorder)
Vulnerability to mental disorders (*see*
  Predisposing factors)

Wages, lost, 159
Waiver of privilege, 182
Waivers for release of confidential
  information, 172
Waiving signature - depositions, 170
War, 9-11, 30, 37-38, 73-87, 114-
  115, 123-124, 138, 142-147
  Civil War, The, 9, 85
  Korean War, 74, 79, 146
  Vietnam conflict, 9-10, 73-87,
    115, 143-144, 146-147
  World War I, 9, 74, 142
  World War II, 9, 78-79, 82, 114,
    146
War experiences (*see* Combat expe-
  riences)
Weapon use - child/adolescent, 45
Weight changes, 68
Withdrawal, 63, 84, 94-95, 98, 101-
    102, 104, 107-108, 110,
    112, 117, 119, 121-123,
    163
  adult SAV, 101-102, 104, 110,
    119, 121-123
  child/adolescent SAV, 94-95, 98,
    107-108, 110, 112, 117
Witness, expert, 167-193
  definition of, 167
  exclusion of, 177-178
  introduction of, 177-178
  preparation of, 187-193
Witnessing atrocities, 11, 25, 83,
    138-141, 143, 147
Work history, 23, 71
Work problems, 68, 124, 150
Work-related accidents, 160, 163
Workers' Compensation Laws, 71,
    157, 159-161, 163
World War I, 9, 74, 142
World War II, 9, 78-79, 82, 114,
    146
Worthlessness, feelings of, 68
Written materials used by expert
  witnesses, 176

**Youth, military - Problems of, 79-
  80, 82**